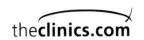

NURSING CLINICS
OF NORTH AMERICA

Sexuality and Chronic Illness:
Assessment and Interventions

GUEST EDITOR
Margaret C. Wilmoth, PhD, MSS, RN

CONSULTING EDITOR
Suzanne S. Prevost, PhD, RN

December 2007 • Volume 42 • Number 4

SAUNDERS

An Imprint of Elsevier, Inc.
PHILADELPHIA   LONDON   TORONTO   MONTREAL   SYDNEY   TOKYO

W.B. SAUNDERS COMPANY
A Division of Elsevier Inc.

1600 John F. Kennedy Blvd., Suite 1800, Philadelphia, PA 19103-2899

http://www.theclinics.com

NURSING CLINICS OF NORTH AMERICA
December 2007
Editor: Ali Gavenda

Volume 42, Number 4
ISSN 0029-6465
ISBN-13: 978-1-4160-5097-1
ISBN-10: 1-4160-5097-3

The ideas and opinions expressed in *Nursing Clinics of North America* do not necessarily reflect those of the Publisher. The Publisher does not assume any responsibility for any injury and/or damage to persons or property arising out of or related to any use of the material contained in this periodical. The reader is advised to check the appropriate medical literature and the product information currently provided by the manufacturer of each drug to be administered to verify the dosage, the method and duration of administration, or contraindications. It is the responsibility of the treating physician or other health care professional, relying on independent experience and knowledge of the patient, to determine drug dosages and the best treatment for the patient. Mention of any product in this issue should not be construed as endorsement by the contributors, editors, or the Publisher of the product or manufacturers' claims.

Nursing Clinics of North America (ISSN 0029-6465) is published quarterly by Elsevier Inc., 360 Park Avenue South, New York, NY 10010-1710. Months of issue are March, June, September, and December. Business and Editorial Offices: 1600 John F. Kennedy Blvd., Suite 1800, Philadelphia, PA 19103-2899. Customer Service Office: 6277 Sea Harbor Drive, Orlando, FL 32887-4800. Periodicals postage paid at New York, NY and additional mailing offices. Subscription price per year is, $123.00 (US individuals), $242.00 (US institutions), $198.00 (international individuals), $290.00 (international institutions), $170.00 (Canadian individuals), $290.00 (Canadian institutions), $65.00 (US students), and $100.00 (international students). To receive student/resident rate, orders must be accompanied by name of affiliated institution, date of term, and the signature of program/residency coordinator on institution letterhead. Orders will be billed at individual rate until proof of status is received. Foreign air speed delivery is included in all *Clinics* subscription prices. All prices are subject to change without notice. **POSTMASTER:** Send address changes to *Nursing Clinics*, Elsevier Periodicals Customer Service, 6277 Sea Harbor Drive, Orlando, FL 32887-4800. **Customer Service: 1-800-654-2452 (US). From outside of the US, call 1-407-345-4000.**

Nursing Clinics of North America is covered in *EMBASE/Excerpta Medica, Index Medicus, Social Sciences Citation Index, Current Contents, ASCA, Cumulative Index to Nursing, RNdex Top 100,* and *Allied Health Literature and International Nursing Index (INI).*

Printed in the United States of America.

CONSULTING EDITOR

SUZANNE S. PREVOST, PhD, RN, Nursing Professor and National HealthCare Chair of Excellence, Middle Tennessee State University, School of Nursing, Murfreesboro, Tennessee

GUEST EDITOR

MARGARET C. WILMOTH, PhD, MSS, RN, Professor, School of Nursing, College of Health and Human Services, University of North Carolina at Charlotte, Charlotte, North Carolina

CONTRIBUTORS

DEBORAH WATKINS BRUNER, RN, PhD, Independence Professor of Nursing Education, School of Nursing; and Director, Recruitment, Retention, and Outreach Core Facility, Abramson Cancer Center, University of Pennsylvania, Philadelphia, Pennsylvania

MARGARET BARTON-BURKE, PhD, RN, Assistant Professor, University of Massachusetts Amherst, Amherst; Nurse Scientist, Yvonne L. Munn Center for Nursing Research, The Institute for Patient Care, Massachusetts General Hospital, Boston; and Associate Clinical Scientist, The Phyllis F. Cantor Center, Dana-Farber Cancer Institute, Boston, Massachusetts

TAMMY CALVANO, MA, Project Manager, School of Nursing, University of Pennsylvania, Philadelphia, Pennsylvania

MATS A.D. CHRISTIANSEN, MNSc, RN, PhD Student, Family Health Care Nursing, University of California, San Francisco; and Assistant Professor, Division of Nursing, Department of Neurobiology, Care Sciences and Society Karolinska Institutet, Huddinge, Sweden

SUZANNE L. DIBBLE, DNSc, RN, Professor Emerita, Institute for Health & Aging, School of Nursing, University of California, San Francisco, San Francisco, California

MICHELE J. ELIASON, PhD, RN, Assistant Professor, Health Education, San Francisco State University, San Francisco, California

TERESA TARNOWSKI GOODELL, PhD, RN, CNS, CCRN, APRN, BC, Assistant Professor, Oregon Health & Science University School of Nursing, Portland, Oregon

CINDY GRANDJEAN, PhD, CANP/GNP, Assistant Professor, The Catholic University of America, Washington, District of Columbia

CAROLYN J. GUSTASON, RN, BSN, OCN, Doctoral Student, Clinical Research Nurse Coordinator II, Cancer Center, Clinical Research Office, University of Massachusetts Medical School, Worcester, Massachusetts

SONYA R. HARDIN, RN, PhD, CCRN, Associate Professor, School of Nursing, University of North Carolina at Charlotte, Charlotte, North Carolina

LINDA U. KREBS, RN, PhD, AOCN, FAAN, Associate Professor, School of Nursing, University of Colorado at Denver and Health Sciences Center, Aurora, Denver, Colorado

LINDA A. MOORE, EdD, APRN, BC (ANP, GNP), MSCN, Associate Professor, School of Nursing, College of Health and Human Services, University of North Carolina at Charlotte; and Nurse Practitioner, Multiple Sclerosis Center, Carolinas Medical Center, Charlotte, North Carolina

BARBARA MORAN, PhD, CNM, FACCE, Assistant Professor, The Catholic University of America, Washington, District of Columbia

ANN MABE NEWMAN, RN, DSN, Associate Professor of Nursing and Adjunct Associate Professor of Women's Studies, School of Nursing, College of Health and Human Services, University of North Carolina at Charlotte, Charlotte, North Carolina

MARIO R. ORTIZ, RN, PhD, APRN, BC, Assistant Professor of Nursing, Purdue University North Central, Westville, Indiana

AMY YRIBARREN POULLOS, BSN, RN, San Carlos, California

RICHARD RICCIARDI, PhD, NP, FAANP, Assistant Professor, Uniformed Services University of the Health Sciences, Bethesda, Maryland; and Chief, Nursing Research Service, Walter Reed Army Medical Center, Washington, District of Columbia

JUDITH A. SHELL, PhD, LMFT, RN, Medical Family Therapist, Marriage and Family Therapist, Osceola Cancer Center, Kissimmee, Florida

CHRISTINA M. SZABO, MS, CNRN, CCRN, Virginia Commonwealth University Health System, Richmond, Virginia

MARGARET C. WILMOTH, PhD, MSS, RN, Professor, School of Nursing, College of Health and Human Services, University of North Carolina at Charlotte, Charlotte, North Carolina

CONTENTS

Nursing is a science and an art. The science aspect of including
sexuality in nursing practice requires knowledge about "normal"
sexual functioning, an understanding of the pathophysiology and
pharmacotherapies that may cause changes in sexuality, and
knowledge about assessing and treating sexual difficulties. The
art of including sexuality into nursing practice comes from
awareness of one's beliefs and values, and comfort in talking
about sexuality. The nurse will find that most patients will be
pleased that he/she has taken the time to broach this important
concern with them. This article provides an overview of the
relationship among sexuality, chronic disease, and quality of life.
Two frameworks are suggested that are useful in operationalizing
sexuality in nursing practice.

It has been well documented that most patients do not volunteer
information about sexual problems, and that health care providers
should incorporate at least a brief sexual assessment into routine
health histories and medical evaluations. While not every nurse
can be a sexual counselor, listening to concerns of patient and
family, presenting factual information in a nonthreatening manner,
managing noncomplex disease and treatment related symptoms,
and providing appropriate referrals can be easily incorporated into
routine care.

congenital or degenerative disease. These individuals experience physical and psychologic consequences that have a profound impact on their sexual health. Using a holistic, developmental, team approach to care, the nurse is well positioned to address the acute and long-term sexual rehabilitation needs of the SCI patient. By assisting SCI patients through the grieving process and promoting a positive, yet realistic, self-concept, nurses can mitigate potential problems in body image disturbances, decreased self-esteem, and gender-specific sexuality issues.

One would think that today's exposure of the topic of sexuality in the electronic and print media would elevate the medical professional's comfort level with communication regarding sexuality issues. However, writers continue to comment on clinician discomfort or lack of discussion with their patients about sexual concerns and anxieties. Many patients want to learn about the implications of their treatment and medications on their sexuality. Nurses who care for chronically ill patients may help foster a more positive self-esteem for the patient, and may influence patient–partner attitudes about worthiness, self-concept, and body image, by providing opportunities to talk about feelings and fears about how treatment may affect their sexuality.

FORTHCOMING ISSUES

RECENT ISSUES

ELSEVIER
SAUNDERS

Nurs Clin N Am 42 (2007) xi–xii

NURSING
CLINICS
OF NORTH AMERICA

Preface

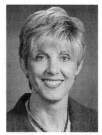

Margaret C. Wilmoth, PhD, MSS, RN
Guest Editor

Sexuality remains an aspect of the human condition that is affected frequently by chronic disease and one that many nurses continue to ignore when providing nursing care. Nurses indicate that the primary reasons why they do not discuss sexuality with their patients are lack of knowledge about sexuality, lack of knowledge about the effects of disease and treatments on sexuality, and discomfort in initiating these conversations. Others say that sexuality is too personal a topic to discuss, while they remain comfortable discussing bowel and bladder habits of their patients.

As members of the most highly respected health profession, nurses are in an enviable position to provide accurate and timely information to our patient populations. Goals of *Healthy People 2010* include reduction of chronic diseases, such as HIV/AIDS, arthritis, and diabetes, and encouraging responsible sexual behavior, implying that nurses must have the latest knowledge about sexuality.

Comments about the lack of readily available knowledge on chronic disease and sexuality are valid, because the last text on sexuality for nurses was published in 1990 [1]. Nursing or medical texts rarely discuss the pathophysiologic implications of disease or treatments on sexuality, and pharmacology texts do not explicitly discuss the impact of medications on sexual functioning. In today's health care environment, practicing nurses do not have time to conduct extensive literature searches on their patients' diagnosis and the impact of treatment on sexuality, despite the fact that they are professionally accountable to address sexuality with their patients.

doi:10.1016/j.cnur.2007.08.009   *nursing.theclinics.com*

This issue of the *Nursing Clinics of North America* intends to rectify this situation by providing nurses with current information on the effects of common chronic diseases and their treatments on sexuality. The approach taken in organizing this issue follows the skills that nurses must posses to include sexuality in their practice. These are communicating about sexuality, knowledge about sexual function in health and illness, and techniques for assessing sexuality. Also included is information about sexuality in populations that often are marginalized by nurses—the gay and lesbian population and those living with HIV/AIDS.

Reading the articles included in this issue will not provide nurses with the final two components key to including sexuality in nursing practice: comfort in talking about sexuality and role models in the work setting who demonstrate this skill. Achieving comfort in talking about sexuality with patients and colleagues can occur by attending conferences, engaging in professional reading, as well as through a journal club format. Role models will emerge as staff engage in dialogue and in education about the chronic illnesses that they commonly see in their setting and when they adopt approaches for sexual assessment for all patients.

It is my hope that you will find this issue informative and provocative for your practice of nursing.

Margaret C. Wilmoth, PhD, MSS, RN
School of Nursing
College of Health and Human Services
University of North Carolina at Charlotte
Charlotte, NC, USA

E-mail address: mcwilmot@uncc.edu

Reference

[1] Fogel CI, Lauver D, editors. Sexual health promotion. Philadelphia: Saunders; 1990.

NURSING
CLINICS
OF NORTH AMERICA

Nurs Clin N Am 42 (2007) 507–514

Sexuality: A Critical Component of Quality of Life in Chronic Disease

Margaret C. Wilmoth, PhD, MSS, RN

School of Nursing, College of Health and Human Services, University of North Carolina at Charlotte, 9201 University City Boulevard, Charlotte, NC 28223, USA

Sexuality and chronic disease are two terms that, on the surface, appear to be diametrically opposed, and yet both have a profound impact on quality of life (QOL). We commonly think of sexuality as being an attribute only for the young and healthy, whereas chronic diseases are experienced primarily by those who are "past their prime" and who, thus, no longer possess the attribute of sexuality, because of age and infirmity. Further complicating the issue is the relative lack of knowledge among health care providers about sexuality in health and illness, and their concomitant lack of comfort in discussing sexuality with their patients. This article defines sexuality and chronic illness and suggests two frameworks that are useful for ensuring that the sexual side effects of chronic disease are addressed by nurses.

Sexuality and chronic disease defined

Sexuality is a complex term that is compounded by having many individual interpretations, with meanings influenced by culture, religion, politics, and other individual factors. The term "sexuality" has not yet been clearly defined in western culture, but one working definition suggests that sexuality is a part of being human and thus, cannot be separated from our humanness and life [1]. As an integral aspect of being human, sexuality is the composite of gender; gender identity and gender roles; sexual orientation; eroticism; pleasure; intimacy; and reproduction of the human race. The ways in which sexuality can be expressed vary as one ages and experiences varying relationships and states of health and illness. It is this expression of sexuality that is often affected by chronic illness (Table 1) [4,9,20–22].

Other terms frequently used interchangeably with sexuality that actually refer to more narrow aspects of this complex construct are sexual

---

E-mail address: mcwilmot@uncc.edu

0029-6465/07/$ - see front matter © 2007 Elsevier Inc. All rights reserved.
doi:10.1016/j.cnur.2007.08.008
nursing.theclinics.com

Table 1
Key definitions

Sexuality	Part of being human; present from birth through death. All that makes us man or woman; perceptions about one's body; the need to touch and connect with others, in both intimate and social settings; interest and ability to engage in sexual behaviors; communication of one's feelings and needs to others; and the ability to engage in satisfying sexual behaviors
Sexual activities	Actions taken to obtain release of sexual tension alone or with another to achieve sexual satisfaction
Sexual behaviors	The multiple ways one verbally and nonverbally communicates sexual feelings and attitudes to others
Sexual functioning	The physiologic component of sexuality, including human sexual anatomy, the sexual response cycle, neuroendocrine functioning, and life-cycle changes in sexual physiology; often affected by pathophysiologic and structural changes to the body and by pharmacologic treatments
Sexual dysfunction	Disturbances in the processes of the sexual response cycle; can be caused by pain associated with sexual intercourse; is a Diagnostic and Statistical Manual for Mental Disorders-IV diagnosis
Sexual response cycle	Two frameworks: Excitement, plateau, orgasm, and resolution Desire, arousal, orgasm
Chronic disease	Prolonged state of ill health without a known cure; may have periods of remission and exacerbation
Quality of life	Ability to enjoy life based on personal goals, values, and beliefs

functioning, sexual activity, and sexual behaviors. These terms typically refer to some aspect of an individual's ability to function physiologically and psychologically; unfortunately, these terms have few uniformly accepted definitions, leaving the meaning up to individual interpretation. Sexual functioning typically refers to an individual's ability to respond to sexual stimulation and to move through the physiologically based sexual response cycle [2]. Sexual activity and sexual behaviors refer to manifestations of sexuality through actions [3]. Sexual dysfunctions as a result of chronic medical conditions are identified in the Diagnostic and Statistical Manual for Mental Disorders-IV [4] and have specific diagnostic criteria that most nurses are not qualified to recognize. Examples of psychiatrically diagnosed sexual dysfunctions include hypoactive sexual desire, dyspareunia, and erectile disorder [4].

The terms "chronic illness" and "chronic disease" are often used interchangeably to describe a structural or functional, pathophysiologic, altered state that lasts longer than 3 months without resolution [5]. Chronic diseases are those illnesses that are prolonged, do not resolve spontaneously, and are rarely cured but may be managed or controlled [5]. According to the US National Center for Health Statistics, nearly one third of all Americans are living with a chronic disease, and it is projected that 50% of the population will be living with at least one chronic disease by 2020 [6].

In addition to the health care costs associated with treating chronic disease are the limitations and disabilities that often result from their diagnosis and treatments. It is these limitations and disabilities that have a negative impact on many aspects of the patient's QOL, which is a complex construct that influences and links the constructs of sexuality and chronic disease. The National Cancer Institute has defined QOL as "the overall enjoyment of life" [7]. QOL is a subjective construct, defined differently by each individual and impacted by factors that vary person to person [8]. Health-related QOL has been proposed as a more distinct aspect of QOL that is often determined to be influenced by health and physical functioning, emotional well-being, social functioning, perceptions about health status, and role functioning capability [8]. Although a full discussion of the constructs of QOL and health-related QOL are beyond the scope of this article, it is important to understand that sexuality is inextricably linked to an individual's subjective appraisal of his/her QOL and thus, should be considered whenever assessing the influence of chronic disease and treatments on QOL (Fig. 1).

Much of chronic disease care uses the concept of symptom in a way that differs from common use. Common use of the term "symptom" is synonymous with the subjective and personal phenomena that commonly accompany the presentation of a clinical problem [9]. When discussing chronic disease care, the side effects of treatments are commonly referred to as symptoms, and the subsequent medical, nursing, and self-care they require are collectively called symptom management [9]. Symptom management has been characterized as a dynamic and multidimensional process that is undertaken to relieve or decrease the distress of a symptom. Most symptoms experienced as a result

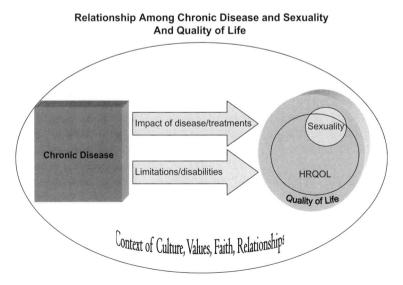

Fig. 1. Relationship among chronic disease, sexuality, and QOL.

of a chronic disease do not occur in isolation, but rather, may occur in a sequential manner or may possibly be interrelated. For example, persons living with either multiple sclerosis or cancer experience profound fatigue that then subsequently may lead to symptoms of depression and a lack of interest in sexual activity. Groups of three or more symptoms that are interrelated are referred to as symptom clusters [10]. It has been suggested that these symptoms may have a negative interactive effect on each other because they affect the patient at the same time. It has also been proposed that this synergy may have a predictive effect on morbidity following treatment [10]. Validation of symptom clusters through research will aid in directing limited resources toward designing innovative interventions for those who suffer from chronic disease. Recognizing that sexuality issues are one of the symptoms experienced as a result of chronic disease, and assisting patients in their understanding and adaptation to these changes, is within the scope of practice of all registered nurses.

Sexuality and nursing responsibility

Sexuality is implicitly and explicitly implied as a component of nursing responsibility by professional nursing organizations. Standards of nursing practice that every nurse is obligated to uphold have been published by the American Nurses Association [11]. The nursing process is identified as the process used in providing holistic care to patients, implying that sexuality is one of the needs to be included in this process of care provision. The Oncology Nursing Society [12] has explicitly identified sexuality as one subject to be included when providing care to cancer patients. Outcomes that patients and their partners are to meet have been identified, and are dependent on the nurse providing information and education about the effects of cancer and its treatment on sexuality. The patient or family

1. Identifies potential or actual changes in sexuality, sexual functioning, or intimacy related to disease and treatment
2. Expresses feelings about alopecia, body image changes, and altered sexual functioning
3. Engages in open communication with his or her partner regarding changes in sexual functioning or desire, within cultural framework
4. Describes appropriate interventions for actual or potential changes in sexual function
5. Identifies other satisfying methods of sexual expression that may provide satisfaction to both partners, within cultural framework
6. Identifies personal and community resources to assist with changes in body image and sexual functioning

Conceptual frameworks

All nurses should have their own theoretic perspective from which they practice and which incorporates the constructs they value into the provision of care. Two examples of conceptual frameworks that may be useful when considering the impact of chronic disease on sexuality are the Johnson Behavioral Systems Model (JBSM) [13] and the Theory of Unpleasant Symptoms (TUS) [14].

The JBSM for Nursing Practice [13,15] is one of the few nursing conceptual frameworks that explicitly identifies sexuality as a major component or subsystem of the human system. Johnson identified eight subsystems that compose man as a behavioral system, one of them being the sexual subsystem. This subsystem has the dual functions of procreation and gratification, which are influenced by biologic sex, gender role identity, and culture [13]. The underlying assumptions of the JBSM include regularity in function, and patterned, repetitive, and purposeful behavior, with the intent of maintaining system integrity. Life stressors and disease leads to temporary or permanent disruption in system functioning. This altered functioning results in some degree of adaptation, manifested by adoption of a new repertoire of behaviors. This new repertoire may be as simple as an increase in pulse, respiration, and blood pressure when confronted by a sudden stressor, or may involve more prolonged behavioral changes, such as loss of fertility and concerns about changes to sexual functioning following a hysterectomy. The JBSM guides patient assessment to determine any challenges in adapting to changes in sexuality and then to analyze more closely the subsystem to identify a nursing diagnosis and select an intervention. The goal is to assist patients in adjusting to behavioral changes so that the subsystem goal is achieved [13].

The TUS [14] is a second framework useful to nurses in their practice. It does not explicitly identify any biopsychosocial subsystems, nor does it specify any disease- or treatment-related symptoms; rather, it describes the characteristics of symptoms and their effect on the individual. The TUS postulates four dimensions to each symptom: intensity, timing, level of distress, and quality. Intensity refers to the strength or severity of the symptom reported by a subject, and is commonly measured by the scores on a self-report measure. Timing includes duration and frequency of occurrence over time, and level of distress is the perception of degree of discomfort. Quality of the symptom experience is a descriptive labeling of the symptom (eg, throbbing versus sharp when describing a pain symptom) [14].

The TUS proposes an iterative relationship and an interrelationship among symptoms and their precursors. Precursors to the symptom include physiologic, psychologic, and situational factors. The symptom experience is proposed to have an effect on the individual, both on daily functioning and on the more global concept of QOL [13]. The TUS is compatible with the Nursing Interventions Classification and Nursing Outcomes Classification and adds assessment dimensions to symptoms that may aid in selecting interventions [14,16,17].

A framework that is useful to consider when beginning incorporating sexuality into discussions with patients is the PLISSIT model [18–22]. The "P" stands for permission, "LI" for limited information, "SS" for specific suggestions, and "IT" for intensive therapy. Simply asking patients about how their disease or medications have affected them sexually is one simple way to let patients know that their sexual concerns are appropriate for them to consider and to discuss with the nurse (permission). Providing limited information to patients about the sexual implications of their diagnosis and treatments is easy to do and can be accomplished when passing medications. More detailed specific suggestions, such as options for sperm banking in an adolescent diagnosed with testicular cancer, requires more time and planning on the part of the nurse. All nurses should be knowledgeable about referral resources in their region for patients needing intensive therapy for either marital or sexual rehabilitation.

Other frameworks are useful in nursing care as it relates to human sexuality, and these are just examples. The key point is that nurses have a professional and ethical, and some might suggest a legal, responsibility to include sexuality in their practice. How this is accomplished composes the art of nursing practice.

Summary

Nursing is a science and an art; one informs the other. The science aspect of including sexuality in nursing practice requires knowledge about "normal" sexual functioning, and an understanding of the pathophysiology and pharmacotherapies that may cause changes in sexuality. The science also includes knowledge about assessing and treating sexual difficulties. The art of including sexuality into nursing practice comes from awareness of one's beliefs, values, and comfort in talking about sexuality. The articles that follow in this issue of *Nursing Clinics of North America* address the science and the art of nursing practice as it relates to including sexuality in your practice. Common chronic diseases and treatments and their associated impact on sexuality are discussed in depth. The art of assessing sexuality and initiating conversations with patients about sexuality are presented. What is left to the reader is to put this new knowledge into practice. Any anxiety the reader might have about talking about sexuality with his/her patients will evaporate the first time he/she asks, "How has your [disease] affected your sexuality and intimate relationships?" The nurse will find that most patients will be pleased that he/she has taken the time to broach this important concern with them.

Further readings

General sexuality resources

American Association of Sex Educators, Counselors and Therapists (AASECT). Ashland, VA. Available at: www.aasect.org/. Accessed August 2, 2007.
Comfort A. The joy of sex: fully revised and completely updated for the 21st century. New York: Octopus Publishing; 2002.

McAnulty RD, Burnette MM. Exploring human sexuality: making healthy decisions. 2nd edition. Boston: Allyn and Bacon; 2007.

Rathus SA, Nevid JS, Richner-Rathus L. Human sexuality in a world of diversity. 6th edition. Boston: A. Pearson Education Company; 2004.

Books on chronic disease with sexuality content

Burke C, editor. Psychosocial nursing guidelines. Pittsburgh (PA): Oncology Nursing Society; 1998.

Dow KH, editor. Nursing care of women and cancer. St. Louis (MO): Mosby; 2006.

Frank-Stromberg M, Olsen SJ, editors. Instruments for clinical health care research. 3rd edition. Philadelphia: Lippincott; 2004.

Katz A. Breaking the silence on cancer and sexuality: a handbook for health care providers. Pittsburgh (PA): Oncology Nursing Society; 2007.

Lubkin IM, Larsen PD, editors. Chronic illness: impact and interventions. 6th edition. Boston: Jones & Bartlett; 2005.

Sipski ML, Alexander CJ. Sexual function in people with disability and chronic illness: a health professional's guide. Rockville (MD): Aspen; 1997.

References

[1] World Health Organization. Department of Reproductive Health and Research (RHR), Working definitions. Available at: http://www.who.int/reproductive-health/gender/ sexual_health.html. Accessed July 17, 2007.

[2] Watts RJ. Sexual functioning, health beliefs and compliance with high blood pressure medications. Nurs Res 1982;31:278–83.

[3] Wilmoth MC, Tingle LR. Development and psychometric testing of the sexual behaviors questionnaire. Can J Nurs Res 2001;32:135–51.

[4] American Psychiatric Association. Diagnostic and statistical manual of mental disorders. 4th edition. Washington (DC): American Psychiatric Association; 1994.

[5] U.S. National Center for Health Statistics. Available at: http://www.cdc.gov/nchs/ VitalStats.htm. Accessed July 24, 2007.

[6] Partnership for Solutions. Available at: http://www.partnershipforsolutions.org. Accessed August 1, 2007.

[7] National Cancer Institute. Available at: www.cancer.gov/Templates/db_alpha.aspx? CdrID=45417. Accessed July 16, 2007.

[8] Abeles RP, Gift HC, Ory MG, editors. Aging and quality of life. New York: Springer; 1994.

[9] Fu MR, LeMone P, McDaniel RW. An integrated approach to an analysis of symptom management in patients with cancer. Oncol Nurs Forum 2004;31(1):65–70.

[10] Dodd MJ, Miaskowski C, Paul SM. Symptom clusters and their effect on the functional status of patients with cancer. Oncol Nurs Forum 2001;28(3):465–70.

[11] American Nurses Association. Nursing scope and standards of practice. Washington, (DC): Author; 2004.

[12] Oncology Nursing Society. Statement on the scope and standards of oncology nursing practice. Pittsburgh (PA): Author; 2004.

[13] Johnson D. The behavioral system model for nursing. In: Riehl JP, Roy C, editors. Conceptual models for nursing practice. New York: Appleton, Century, Crofts; 1980. p. 207–16.

[14] Lenz ER, Pugh LC, Milligan RA, et al. The middle-range theory of unpleasant symptoms: an update. Advances in Nursing Science 1997;19(3):14–27.

[15] Grubbs J. An interpretation of the Johnson Behavioral System Model for nursing practice. In: Riehl JP, Roy C, editors. Conceptual models for nursing practice. New York: Appleton, Century, Crofts; 1980. p. 217–54.

[16] McCloskey JC, Bulechek GM, editors. Nursing interventions classification (NIC). 3rd edition. St. Louis (MO): Mosby; 2000.

[17] Moorhead S, Johnson M, Maas M, editors. Nursing outcomes classification (NOC). 3rd edition. St. Louis (MO): Mosby; 2004.

[18] Annon JS. The behavioral treatment of sexual problems. Honolulu (Hawaii): Mercantile Printing; 1974.

[19] Wilmoth MC. Sexuality. In: Lubkin IM, Larsen PD, editors. Chronic illness: impact and interventions. 6th edition. Boston: Jones and Bartlett; 2006. p. 285–304.

[20] Wilmoth MC. Sexuality. In: Burke C, editor. Psychosocial dimensions of oncology nursing care. Pittsburgh (PA): Oncology Nursing Press; 1998. p. 102–27.

[21] Masters WH, Johnson VE. Human sexual response. Philadelphia: Lippincott-Raven; 1966.

[22] Kaplan HS. The new sex therapy: active treatment of sexual dysfunctions. New York: Brunner/Mazel, Publishers; 1974.

NURSING CLINICS
OF NORTH AMERICA

Nurs Clin N Am 42 (2007) 515–529

Sexual Assessment: Research and Clinical

Linda U. Krebs, RN, PhD, AOCN, FAAN

School of Nursing, University of Colorado at Denver and Health Sciences Center, Aurora, C288-18, 4200 East Ninth Avenue, Denver, CO 80262, USA

Sexuality is an important part of the total person and is integral to the overall health, quality of life, and general well being of every individual [1]. Although not always accurately portrayed, sexuality is more than the act of intercourse. It includes intimacy, touching, a multitude of activities to show affection, and a variety of methods to communicate with others. Chronic disease and treatment may disrupt or permanently alter one's ability to maintain previous sexual patterns; however, disease or disability cannot alter the fact that one is a sexual being [2].

Human sexuality as a concept defies easy definition, in part because the distinction between sex and sexuality are not often or easily made. According to Schover [3], "Sexuality includes more than erections or orgasms. It includes feeling attractive and lovable (relational sex), feeling free to enjoy touch and caressing (recreational sex), having functional sexual activity and being able to have children if desired (reproductive sex)" [3]. The Pan American Health Organization [4] defines sex as "the sum of biological characteristics that define the spectrum of humans as females and males" [4] and sexuality as "a core dimension of being human which includes sex, gender, sexual and gender identity, sexual orientation, eroticism, emotional attachment/love, and reproduction. ... (and) is a result of the interplay of biological, psychological, socioeconomic, cultural, ethical and religious/spiritual factors" [4]. The World Health Organization [5] defines sexuality as one of the "central aspects of being human" [5], and Magnan [6] notes that "sexual health and issues related to human sexuality are becoming increasingly important areas of concern for healthcare professionals both nationally and globally" [6].

Sexual dysfunction is often multifactorial, including a variety of physical, psychologic, and sociocultural factors [7]. Chronic medical conditions are

E-mail address: Linda.krebs@uchsc.edu

frequently associated with sexual difficulties and problems which are often underreported and underdiagnosed [8]. Some individuals are at higher risk for sexual side effects than others based on age, gender, type of disease or disability, type of treatment, or concomitant medical or psychologic illness [2,9,10]. Patients deserve the opportunity to have their sexual problems appropriately and thoughtfully identified and addressed [2].

Components of a sexual assessment

An effective sexual assessment consists of a variety of models, discussion questions, and evaluation instruments that can accurately and adequately assess the patient's potential and actual areas of sexual dysfunction. The assessment may be brief or intensive, covering such topics as sexual activity, intimacy, communication patterns, current relationships, disease and treatment issues, satisfaction with current activities, and coping skills. Additional topics, based on the identified, individual needs of the patient and partner, that may be incorporated into a sexual assessment as needed or appropriated include [11–16]:

Frequency and type of sexual activities	Social support network
Premorbid, baseline and follow-up levels of sexual function and satisfaction	Disability history including disability-related symptoms
History of sexual activity with men, women, both and number of current sexual partners	History of sexual trauma, rape or domestic abuse
Cognitive function	Use of contraception and safe sex practices
Previous vaccinations (hep A/B, HPV)	Reproductive status and desire for future childbearing
Previous testing (HIV/Hep/Syphillis)	

Nusbaum [16] suggests a general approach that includes evaluating one's own attitudes and beliefs about sexuality, being sensitive and nonjudgmental, avoiding medical jargon, identifying patient and partner concerns, obtaining a thorough medical history, evaluating psychosocial and psychosexual issues, exploring intervention options, and promoting safe sex.

Sexual assessment in chronic illness

As previously identified, those with chronic illness or disability are likely to experience sexual dysfunction related to illness, treatment, or a combination of both, as well as to psychologic factors or relationship factors that may influence sexual function. Any of these factors can result in altered body image, decreased self-esteem, an inability to take part in usual sexual activities, or changes in procreation abilities which may lead to various levels of dysfunction [2,9]. Common chronic illnesses are often associated with decreased libido, alterations in desire and arousal, decreased or absent ejaculation and orgasm, and may be associated with pain, fatigue, depression, and decreased movement and mobility, any of which may impact sexuality and sexual function [7,17–22].

Before beginning any assessment, nurses must have at least a rudimentary understanding of the potential sexual side effects related to the diseases and disabilities most commonly seen and the treatments most commonly prescribed within their workplace settings. Table 1 denotes the potential sexual side effects seen with some common chronic conditions, while Table 2 [23–25] identifies potential medical, psychologic, and relationship factors that may impact sexuality and sexual function. Even though many diagnoses and treatments have the potential to cause sexual dysfunction, the level of dysfunction and the patient's reaction to it will vary with each individual. It is essential that assessment and eventual interventions are based on the specific issues, concerns, and needs of the patient (and partner, as appropriate).

Sexual assessment models

A number of models have been developed to assess current sexual function (ALARM [26], Schover [27]), with additional models, primarily focused on providing interventions to manage sexual dysfunction, that can also be used for assessment before intervention (PLISSIT [28], Ex-PLISSIT [29,30], BETTER [31]). Most assessment models evaluate levels of sexual activity, arousal and lubrication, ability to reach orgasm, and resolution following orgasm. These models also evaluate disease and disability, treatment and side effect status, and comorbidities, and include current medications (prescribed, over the counter, and complementary) [26,27]. The models developed for intervention either assume that the nurse has adequately assessed the level of sexual dysfunction before identifying interventions, or allows the nurse to both assess and intervene concomitantly [28–31]. The most commonly used model is the PLISSIT (permission, limited information, specific suggestions, intensive therapy) model first described by Annon in 1974 [28]. This model includes giving the patient permission to discuss sexuality issues and to be sexually active, provides limited information that will explain potential side effects, expands to providing specific suggestions based on specific patient or partner-derived concerns, and includes the use of intensive therapy by trained sex counselors for those needing interventions beyond the scope of the nurse. An extension of this model, Ex-PLISSIT, developed by Davis and Tyler, incorporates permission-giving at each level, as well as specific discussion review with the patient and partner, and reflection on the interaction by the provider to enhance professional or personal knowledge and growth [29]. An additional model, BETTER (bring up; explain, tell, time, educate, record), developed by Mick and colleagues [31], incorporates the need to bring up the topic of

Table 1
Potential sexual dysfunction based on diagnosis or disability

Diagnosis	Potential sexual dysfunction
Cancer	Decreased libido
	Problems with maintaining an erection/ejaculation
	Difficulty with arousal/lubrication
	Decreased frequency of sexual activity
	Infertility
	Dyspareunia
	Decreased sexual satisfaction
	Early menopause/menopausal symptoms
Chronic obstructive pulmonary disease	Decreased libido/arousal
	Erectile dysfunction
	Decreased ability for sexual function caused by sob and hypoxia
Coronary artery disease/ myocardial infarction	Reduced frequency of sexual activity
	Fear of angina, new myocardial infarction
	Erectile dysfunction
	Decreased arousal
	Concomitant depression
	Decreased sexual satisfaction
Diabetes	Decreased libido/arousal
	Erectile dysfunction
	Retrograde ejaculation
	Chronic vulvovaginal candidosis
Hypertension	Erectile dysfunction
	Decreased arousal
Multiple sclerosis	Decreased libido
	Retrograde ejaculation
	Delayed or absent orgasm
Parkinson's disease	Libido may be increased due to dopaminergic medications but generally decreased libido, particularly in women
	Retrograde ejaculation
Renal failure	Decreased libido
	Erectile dysfunction
	Annovulation
	Amenorrhea
Spinal cord injury	Erectile dysfunction
	Decreased lubrication
	Delayed/absent ejaculation
	Delayed or absent orgasm

Data from Refs. [7,17–22].

sexuality, evaluate and explain current activities and beliefs, and concludes with the essential component of providing a written report and plan in the patient's chart so that others may continue the discussion and intervention. Table 3 provides a brief overview of all five models, including their primary use for either assessment or intervention.

Table 2
Overview of medical and psychosocial effects of disease on sexual function

Medical factors	Psychological factors	Relationship factors
Disease or treatment symptoms and side effects (eg, pain, fatigue, nausea)	Fear of triggering new myocardial infarcton or cerebrovascular accident	Communication difficulties
Mobility limitations	Fear of causing hurt or harm	Lack of intimacy, trust
Alterations in physical sensations (eg, burning, hypersensitivity, itching)	Altered body image and self-esteem	Partner's reaction to illness
Alterations in ability to ejaculate, reach orgasm	Fear of rejection by partner	Partner's personal sexual dysfunction
Dyspnea or angina upon sexual stimulation	Preoccupation with disease or treatment	Cultural and societal beliefs
Altered body function/body image (eg, ostomy, disfigurement, alopecia)	Limited coping skills	Lack of privacy (eg, when hospitalized, in a care facility)
Comorbidities (eg, arthritis, diabetes, chronic obstructive pulminary disease)	Past physical, sexual, emotional abuse	Alterations in social, work, family, or marital role
Medications (for treatment, side effects, other illnesses)	Pre-existing patterns of sexual behaviors, attitudes and beliefs	Inability to meet or find a partner
		Quality of partnered relationship

Data from Refs. [17,23–25].

Assessment methods

Most health care providers involved in sexual assessment focus on one of two methods to evaluate current sexual status and concerns: a brief assessment or a more in-depth, intensive assessment [15,32]. The decision of which method to select is based most often on time available for assessment, potential level of dysfunction, patient identified concerns, and the comfort, skill, and knowledge level of the health care provider. The first step in either method is to normalize and legitimize the discussion of sexuality, highlighting the importance of accurately assessing beliefs and concerns about sexuality and sexual function while making the discussion a normal part of a routine nursing or medical assessment. Comments such as, "I usually ask about sexuality and sexual function with everyone diagnosed with [the patient's diagnosis] or who will be treated with [medication that may affect sexual function]" will normalize and legitimize the nurse's discussion of this sensitive topic [2,9,33]. Then, while focusing on the areas outlined in standard assessment models, the brief assessment method asks a few short questions that allows the nurse to open the topic and assess current concerns.

Table 3
Models for assessment or intervention

ASSESSMENT (Primary)		INTERVENTION (Primary); ASSESSMENT (Secondary)		
ALARM model (Anderson & Lamb, 1995)	Schover method (Schover, 1998)	PLISSIT (Annon, 1974)	Extended PLISSIT (Ex-PLISSIT) (Davis & Taylor, 2006)	BETTER (Mick, Hughes, & Cohen, 2004)
A - Activity (sexual) L - Libido/desire (level/existence of) A - Arousal/orgasm (ability to attain) R - Resolution/release/relaxation (ability to attain) M - Medical information (current, past, and concomitant health status; medications)	Evaluate past and present: Sexual activities Sexual functioning Sexual relationships Evaluate current: Disease or disability Treatment Comorbidities Psychological status Coping skills Identify sexual goals, desires and knowledge	P - Permission (to have sexual feelings and relationships) LI - Limited Information (about treatment/disease/disability on sexuality) SS - Specific Suggestions (to manage sexual side effects) IT - Intensive Therapy (1st three can usually be accomplished by the health care provider, the last may require referral to sex therapist or counselor)	Uses the 4 stage PLISSIT model Permission giving is a core component of all stages. All interactions are reviewed with the patient at the time of assessment and at future assessments. Reflection is incorporated into each stage to challenge the nurse's assumptions and enhance self-awareness P – allows for identification of potential issues now and in the future LI – allows nurse to dispel myths, correct misconceptions, give factual information limited to what the patient needs SS – addresses all aspects of sexuality and sexual health (not just behavior); suggestions are tailored to meet the individual's needs IT – identify services and refer as appropriate	Bring up issues of sexuality/sexual function Explain that sexuality is integral to QOL and important to discuss Tell patients that resources are available and provide assistance to obtain those needed Timing is crucial; discussions should be facilitated as the patient/partner desires Educate the patient/partner about potential/expected changes in sexuality and sexual function Record discussions, assessments, interventions and outcomes in the patient's health care record

Abbreviation: QOL, quality of life.
Data from Refs. [26–31].

Questions that might be asked focus on current relationships, who these are with (men, women, or both), and whether there are any concerns (for patient or partner) or any symptoms, such as pain or fatigue. For the person without a relationship, the focus will be on sexual concerns or on issues that may have contributed to a lack of sexual behavior [15,32].

For a more intensive assessment, most believe that a combination of direct and open-ended questions should be included [34]. Direct questions, such as those used in the brief assessment, can start the initial discussion, while open-ended questions allow for more in-depth understanding of concerns. Questions can be asked regarding beliefs about intimacy, types of sexual activities preferred, relationships, specific alterations related to disease or treatment, or anything else that will provide insight into patient issues and concerns. In the 1980s, Woods [35] identified potential sexual assessment questions that are still pertinent today, while more recent authors have expanded upon these questions to increase the scope and depth of the assessment [2,6,34,36–40]. Potential questions include:

How has your diagnosis/treatment affected the way you see yourself as a man/woman/sexual being; wife/husband/partner?

What aspects of your sexuality do you believe have been affected by your diagnosis/treatment (include both positive and negative)?

How often do you engage in sexual activities? Is this normal/usual for you? Are you satisfied with this?

How often do you experience a spontaneous desire for sex?

How easy is it for you to feel subjective pleasure with sexual stimulation? What type of stimulation is needed to achieve orgasm?

How much do you know about current aspects of your disease/treatment/ other planned interventions?

Do you have any questions about sexuality or sexual activity?

Are you satisfied with your sexual response (erection, including firmness; orgasm, lubrication, etc.)?

Do you participate in oral sex? Anal sex?

Do you or your partner use any devices or substances to increase sexual pleasure?

What information, interventions, or resources can I provide to help you fulfill your sexuality?

How important is sexual intimacy to you?

Have you talked with your partner about your feelings?

More in-depth, intensive assessments may also include the use of one or more questionnaires, inventories, or surveys that assess sexual beliefs and values, ability to function, and sexual satisfaction (Table 4) [41–43]. While use of these instruments may be extremely valuable in facilitating a complete, accurate assessment, they should be used to complement but not supplant clinical judgment.

Table 4
Instruments to assess sexuality or sexual function

General (male and female, generic sexuality):

Instrument	Abbreviation	Items
Changes in sexual functioning questionnaire	CSFQ	Females = 35 items; Males = 36 items; Self-report = 14 items
Derogatis interview for sexual functioning	DISF/DISF-SR	25 items
Derogotis sexual functioning inventory	DSFI	254 items
Sex history form	SHF	46 items
Watts sexual function questionnaire	WSFQ	17 items
Men (general sexuality, erectile dysfunction, lower urinary tract issues):		
Brief sexual functioning inventory	BMSFI	11 items
Center for marital and sexual Health sexual function questionnaire	CMSH-SFQ	Baseline = 17 items; Follow-up = 23 items
International index of erectile dysfunction	IIEF	15 items
Male sexual health questionnaire	MSHQ	25 items
Sexual health inventory for men (modified from IIEF)	SHIM	5 items
Sexual function index (SFI, 11 items)	SFI	11 items
Women (general sexuality, desire, satisfaction):		
Brief index of sexual functioning for women	BISF-W	22 items
Female sexual function	FSFI	19 items
Golombuk-Rusk inventory of sexual satisfaction	GRISS	28 items
Self-perception of female sexuality	SPFS	123 items
Wilmoth sexual behaviors questionnaire-female	WSBQ-F	54 items

Adapted from Refs. [10,21,41–45].

Barriers to assessment

Much has been written about the need to accurately and adequately assess all patients for sexual complications related to disease and treatment [11,15,16,32,40,44]. Regardless of the identified need, most research shows that there are significant barriers to sexual assessment [2,9,22,32,33,36, 44–49]. Many health care providers rarely discuss sexual concerns, citing a variety of personal and professional reasons. Those most commonly cited include personal discomfort, lack of training or knowledge, and fears of embarrassing themselves or their patients. For nurses, the most common barriers identified include lack of time, heavy workload, inadequate training, and the belief that talking about sexuality is not an expected component of the nurse's role [6,36,49]. One of the most frequently cited concerns is the fear of "opening a can of worms, opening the floodgates, or opening Pandora's box." This is in reference to gaining information the nurse is not prepared to deal with because of inadequate knowledge and expertise, because he or she does not have adequate personal or professional resources to manage, or which could increase the patient's anxiety or distress while potentially opening the nurse to legal or professional liability [49]. Of specific concern is addressing sensitive topics, such as sexuality, with those who are older or those of a different gender, race or ethnicity, culture or sexual orientation, or who primarily speak a different language from the nurse. In addition, numerous other barriers have been identified and include: lack of privacy; personal or societal beliefs about acceptability of being sexually active in times of illness, disability, or old age; being unclear about the appropriate language or words to use; and a multitude of fears, such as the fear of negative reactions from peers, being unable to cope with issues raised by the patient or partner, or that addressing the issue is inappropriate to the current health care situation [2,9,22,32,33,36,44-49].

Strategies to assure a comprehensive, accurate assessment

Strategies to improve sexual assessment include those that affect the nurse–patient interaction, as well as those that will decrease the barriers to nurse instigation of a discussion of sexuality and sexual function with the patient or partner. Nurse–patient interaction strategies focus on communication (style and context), environment, sociocultural beliefs and values, and content and timing. Strategies to decrease nurse barriers to conducting the assessment focus on the nurse's knowledge and skill, level of comfort and confidence, and the use of standards and guidelines to direct practice.

Having knowledge, training, and practical experience to assess sexual concerns are essential components of conducting an accurate and appropriate sexual assessment, but in and of themselves, they are insufficient. In order for nurses to provide an accurate assessment, even if the assessment is brief or is conducted only to gather information before referring the patient onto a more competent provider, they must first understand their own sexual identity and what constitutes personally acceptable sexual patterns and practices. Nurses also must have an understanding of the potential psychosocial, sociocultural, environmental, and medical aspects that may impact sexual function for this specific patient. Being comfortable with one's own sexuality as well as having basic knowledge about sexual issues and concerns will facilitate the assessment and should allow the nurse to carry out the assessment with a nonjudgmental and caring approach [2,11,44,50].

Strategies to assure accurate, comprehensive assessments

While many patients may have sexual concerns, most will not broach the subject with the health care provider for fear that it is an inappropriate topic, because of the potential for embarrassment, and the need to place the primary focus on disease or disability management [47–49]. Thus, asking the patient about sexuality as part of the clinical assessment and throughout medical visits or hospital admissions legitimizes and normalizes the subject and gives patients permission to discuss sexual issues. The patient's current sexual practices, cultural and religious beliefs, relationships, communication patterns, and general intimacy issues should be incorporated into the discussion. Additionally, the patient's partner should be included whenever possible and appropriate, and always with the patient's permission. It is essential to avoid medical jargon and value oriented terminology, and to speak in a straightforward, matter of fact, professional manner, with confidence and without embarrassment. Questions should be gender neutral. For cultures where it is acceptable, maintain eye contact and sit rather than stand. The suggested framework for the assessment is to proceed from less sensitive to more sensitive issues, and to continually clarify responses to assure accurate understanding of both verbal and nonverbal communication. Questions and responses should acknowledge the subject and related concerns as being normal and important. Additionally, the focus should be on the specific concerns of the patient and partner. If it becomes clear that the scope of concerns or specific issues raised by the patient and partner are beyond the capability of the nurse, a referral to an appropriate, licensed therapist for further assessment and intervention should be provided [2,9,22,32,33,36,44–49,51,52].

The initial discussion should start with the assumption that patients have some level of sexual knowledge and experience. Timing of the assessment is essential. Establishing rapport and gaining a level of trust will enhance the discussion. The assessment should not be conducted as if one was going down a laundry list of questions, but rather the answers to one question should lead to next question or area for discussion. Bridge statements, that move the discussion from one topic to the next, should be used and terminology should be understandable and comfortable for the patient [2,6,9,11,15,32,33,36,44,49,53].

Strategies to increase nurse knowledge and comfort

Integrating the topic of sexuality and sexual dysfunction into practice requires many skills that most nurses do not obtain in basic nursing education, and may not have access to through their place of employment. While many nursing programs do include some information on sexuality, sexual health, and potential sexual dysfunction related to various diseases or treatments, the majority of content is presented during the student's assessment classes at the same time the student is trying to learn basic skills necessary for initial clinical experiences. Trying to incorporate discussions about sensitive topics at the same time the student is trying to master basic skills may relegate the topic of sexual dysfunction to a "nice but not necessary to know at this time" status. Additionally, for the student to begin incorporation of appropriate techniques in assessing sexuality issues, there need to be role models, usually in the form of clinical faculty. Unfortunately, many clinical faculty have not had either the experience or training, nor mastered comfort and confidence, in these activities to be effective role models [2,9,22,32,33,36,44–49]. Participating in continuing education programs, either online or in person, and in journal clubs focused on sexually-related issues and the use of role models can provide the novice nurse with initial skills for sexual assessment. Additional skills can be gained through continual incorporation of sexuality assessment and counseling into daily nursing practice, role playing, attending advanced seminars, taking part in values clarification exercises, and participating in interdisciplinary rounds and educational offerings. The most valuable educational offerings include cognitive (theory and research), affective (small group interaction and values clarification), and communication components of learning, as well as experiential activities that allow the participant to practice techniques that may decrease embarrassment and fear [2,9,22,32,33,36,44–49,51,52].

Places of employment can develop standards or guidelines for sexual assessment, as well as be sure that sexual health questions are incorporated into nursing admission databases. Additionally, work settings can support nurses in conducting sexual assessments by offering additional education or encouraging nurses to pursue outside opportunities, providing resources or access to resources for referrals once sexual concerns have been identified, or through adhering to the principle that assisting patients and their partners with sexual alterations is congruent with and integral to the nurse's role in providing holistic care [2,11,44].

Nursing research

The potential for nursing research in the areas of sexuality and sexual function assessment are vast. While literature exits about physician barriers to assessment, few definitive studies exist in relation to nurse barriers and methods to overcome these barriers. Specific strategies that may facilitate the assessment process, including the use of diaries and other methods to monitor sexual function [54] need to be developed and studies conducted; while specific methods to enhance the knowledge and expertise of nurses who will conduct assessments need to be evaluated and incorporated into various levels of nursing education. Finally, additional nurse-designed assessment models and evaluation instruments need to be developed and validated with specific disease and culturally-specific patient populations [55].

Summary

It has been well documented that most patients do not volunteer information about sexual problems and that health care providers should incorporate at least a brief sexual assessment into routine health histories and medical evaluations. Opening the door to a discussion on current or potential alterations in sexuality and sexual function is often met with relief by the patient and partner who are unsure if sexuality is a relevant topic in the brief encounter with a health care provider. Penson believes that "it is incumbent upon the health care providers to give patients the opportunity to discuss the issues of sexuality and sexual functioning associated with their specific disease and treatment" [34]. While not every nurse can be a sexual counselor, listening to concerns of patient and family, presenting factual information in a nonthreatening manner, managing noncomplex disease and treatment-related symptoms, and providing appropriate referrals can be easily incorporated into routine care. Assisting patients with sexual alterations is congruent with, integral to, and an essential component of the nurse's role in providing holistic care [2].

Resources

The following resources may assist the nurse in understanding potential alterations in sexuality and sexual function, appropriate methods of assessment, and in identifying potential interventions. Some require a search of the site using the key words "sexuality" or "sexual dysfunction."

In general, health care professionals should consider the following list of points when considering opening the door to discussing sexuality in the medical setting:

- Sexuality and sexual health are integral to quality of life and overall health.

Organization	Website
American Association of Sex Educators, Counselors and Therapists (AASECT)	http://www.aasect.org
CancerBACUP	http://www.cancerbacup.org.uk
Healthfinder	http://healthfinder.gov
Mayo Clinic	http://www.mayoclinic.com
MedlinePlus	http://www.nlm.nih.gov/medlineplus/medlineplus.html
National Cancer Institute	http://cancernet.nci.nih.gov
National Institute on Aging	http://www.niapublications.org/agepages/sexuality.asp
National Institute of Diabetes and Digestive and Kidney Diseases	http://www.niddk.nih.gov/health/health.htm
Sexual Functioning Advisory Council of the American Foundation for Urologic Disease	http://www.afud.org
Sex Information and Education Council	http://www.siecus.org
The Sexual Health Network: Sex Therapy, Expert Education	http://www.sexualhealth.com
Women's Health America	http://www.womenshealth.com

- Patients deserve the opportunity to discuss their sexual concerns with a qualified health care professional.
- Sexual assessments should occur at the time of initial patient interactions, throughout treatment and during follow-up.
- Models and evaluation tools are available to facilitate assessments.
- Comprehensive assessments require sensitivity, caring, knowledge, skill and timing.
- Appropriately educated nurses are well qualified to conduct sexual assessments and to provide options for interventions and referrals.

References

[1] Nusbaum MRH, Gamble G, Skinner B, et al. The high prevalence of sexual concerns among women seeking routine gynecological care. J Fam Pract 2000;49(3):229–32.

[2] Krebs LU. Sexual and reproductive dysfunction. In: Yarbro C, Frogge MH, Goodman M, Groenwald S, editors. Cancer nursing: principles and practice. 6th edition. Boston: Jones and Bartlett; 2005. p. 841–69.

[3] Schover LR. Addressing the sexual needs of cancer survivors. Presented at the 9th Biennial Symposium on Minorities, the Medically Underserved & Cancer. Washington, DC, March 24, 2004.

[4] Pan American Health Organization, World Health Organization. Promotion of Sexual Health. Available at: http://www2.hu-berlin.de/sexology/GESUND/ARCHIV/PSH.HTM. Accessed on May 23, 2007.

[5] WHO. What constitutes sexual health? Prog Reprod Health Res [serial online] 2004;67:2–3. Available at: http://www.who.int/reproductive-health/hrp/progress/67.pdf. Accessed on May 23, 2007.

[6] Magnan M, Reynolds K. Barriers to addressing patient sexuality concerns across five areas of specialization. Clin Nurse Spec 2006;20(6):285–92.

[7] Nusbaum MRH, Hamilton C, Lenahan P. Chronic illness and sexual functioning. Am Fam Physician 2003;67(2):347–54, 357.

[8] Bitzer J, Platano G, Tschudin S, et al. Sexual counseling for women in the context of physical diseases: a teaching model for physicians. J Sex Med 2007;4(1):29–37.

[9] Krebs LU. Sexuality and reproductive issues. In: Yasko J, editor. Nursing management of symptoms associated with chemotherapy. 5th edition. Philadelphia: Meniscus; 2001. p. 205–14.

[10] National Cancer Institute. Sexuality and reproductive issues (PDQ®) health professional issue. Available at:http://www.cancer.gov/cancertopics/pdq/supportivecare/sexuality/health professional/. Accessed on May 23, 2007.

[11] Katz A. Do ask, do tell. Am J Nurs 2005;105(7):66–8.

[12] Cristian A. The assessment of the older adult with a physical disability: a guide for clinicians. Clin Geriatr Med 2006;22:221–38.

[13] Jones R, Bartob S. Introduction to history taking and principles of sexual health. Postgrad Med J 2004;80:444–6.

[14] Nusbaum MRH, Lenahan P, Sadovsky R. Sexual health in aging men and women. Geriatrics 2005;60(9):18–23.

[15] Nusbaum MRH, Hamilton CD. The proactive sexual health history. Am Fam Physician 2002;66(9):1705–12.

[16] Nusbaum MRH, Lanahan P, Sadovsky R. Addressing the physiologic and psychological sexual changes that occur with age. Geriatrics 2005;60(9):18–23.

[17] Basson R, Schultz WW. Sexual sequelae of general medical disorders. Lancet 2007;369: 409–24.

[18] Johnson BK. Prostate cancer and sexuality: implications for nursing. Geriatr Nurs 2004; 25(6):341–7.

[19] Carmack Taylor CL, Basen-Enquist K, Shinn EH, et al. Predictors of sexual functioning in ovarian cancer patients. J Clin Orthod 2004;2295:881–9.

[20] Sumanen M, Ojanlatva A, Koskenvuo M, et al. GPs should discuss sex life issues with coronary patients. Sexual and Rehabilitation Therapy 2005; 20(4):443–52.

[21] Matzaroglou C, Assimakopoulos K, Panagiotopoulous E, et al. Sexual function in females with severe cervical spinal cord injuries: a controlled study with the Female Sexual Function Index. Int J Rehabil Res 2005; 28(4):375–77.

[22] Katz A. Sexuality and myocardial infarction. Am J Nurs 2007;107(3):49–52.

[23] Stausmire JM. Sexuality at the end of life. Am J Hosp Palliat Care 2004;21:33–9.

[24] Ganz PA, Desmond KA, Belin TR, et al. Predictors of sexual health in women after a breast cancer diagnosis. J Clin Oncol 1999;17:2371–80.

[25] Nusbaum MRH, Singh AR, Pyles AA. Sexual healthcare needs of women aged 65 and older. J Am Geriatr Soc 2004;52:117–22.

[26] Andersen BL, Lamb M. Sexuality and cancer. In: Murphy GP, Lawrence W, Lenhard RE, editors. American Cancer Society textbook of clinical oncology. 2nd edition. Atlanta (GA): American Cancer Society; 1995. p. 699–713.

[27] Schover LR. Sexual dysfunction. In: Holland JC, editor. Psycho-oncology. New York: Oxford University Press; 1998. p. 494–9.

[28] Annon JS. The behavioral treatment of sexual problems. Honolulu (HI): Mercantile Printing; 1974. p. 43–7.

[29] Davis S, Taylor B. From PLISSIT to Ex-PLISSIT. In: Davis S, editor. Rehabilitation: the use of theories and models in practice. Edinburgh: Elsevier; 2006. p. 101–29.

[30] Taylor B, Davis S. Using the extended PLISSIT model to address sexual healthcare needs. Nurs Stand 2006;21(11):35–40.

[31] Mick J, Hughes M, Cohen MZ. Using the BETTER model to assess sexuality. Clin J Oncol Nurs 2004;8(1):84–6.

[32] Kingsberg SA. Taking a sexual history. Obstet Gynecol Clin 2006;33:535–47.

[33] Krebs LU. Cancer 101: I don't know what to say: Talking with your patients about sexuality issues. Clin J Oncol Nurs 2006;10(3):313–5.

[34] Penson RT, Gallagher J, Gioiella ME, et al. Sexuality and cancer: conversation comfort zone. Oncologist 2000;5:336–44.

[35] Woods NF. Human sexuality in health and illness. St. Louis (MO): CV Mosby; 1984.

[36] Magnan M, Reynolds KE, Galvin EA. Barriers to addressing patient sexuality in nursing practice. Medsurg Nurs 2005;14(5):282–9.

[37] Warner PH, Rowe T, Whipple B. Shedding light on the sexual history. Am J Nurs 1999; 99(6):34–40.

[38] Wallace M. Sexuality. Medsurg Nurs 2004;13(2):122–3.

[39] McKee AL, Schover LR. Sexuality rehabilitation. Cancer 2001;92(4):1008S–12S.

[40] Ohl LE. Essentials of female sexual dysfunction from a sex therapy perspective. Urol Nurs 2007;27(1):57–63.

[41] Cappelleri JC, Rosen RC. The sexual health inventory for men (SHIM): a 5-year review of research and clinical experience. Int J Impot Res 2005;17:307–19.

[42] Creti L, Fichten CS, Amsel R, et al. "Global Sexual Functioning:" A single summary score for Nowinksi and LoPiccolo's Sexual History Form (SHF). In: Davis CM, Yarber WL, Bauserman R, Schreer G, Davis SL, editors. Handbook of sexuality-related measures. Thousand Oaks (CA): Sage Publications; 1998. p. 261–7.

[43] PROQOLID (the Patient-reported Outcome and Quality of Life Instruments Database). Sexuality. Available at: http://www.qolid.org/proqolid/layout/set/print/search_1/pathologydisease?pty=1926. Accessed on May 23, 2007.

[44] Albaugh JA, Kellogg-Spadt S. Sexuality and sexual health: The nurse's role and initial approach to patients. Urol Nurs 2003;23(3):227–8.

[45] Katz A. Sexuality after hysterectomy: a review of the literature and discussion of nurse' role. J Adv Nurs 2003;42(3):297–303.

[46] Rosen R, Kountz D, Post-Zwicker T, et al. Sexual communication skills in residency training: the Robert Wood Johnson model. J Sex Med 2006;3(1):37–46.

[47] Gott M, Hinchliff S. Barriers to seeking treatment for sexual problems in primary care: a qualitative study with older people. Fam Pract 2003;20(6):690–5.

[48] Gott M, Hinchliff S, Galena E. General practitioner attitudes to discussing sexual health issues with older people. Soc Sci Med 2004;58:2093–103.

[49] Gott M, Galena E, Hinchliff S, Elford H. "Opening a can of worms": GP and practice nurse barriers to talking about sexual health in primary care. Fam Pract 2004;21(5):528–36.

[50] Wilmoth MC, Bruner DB. Integrating sexuality into cancer nursing practice. Oncology Nursing: Patient Treatment and Support 2002;9(1):1–14.

[51] Bickford B. Sexual history taking and genital examination. Primary Health Care 2006;16(2): 33–5.

[52] Dattilo J, Brewer MK. Assessing clients' sexual health as a component of holistic nursing practice. J Holist Nurs 2005;23(2):208–19.

[53] Maughan K, Clarke C. The effect of a clinical nurse specialist in gynaecological oncology on quality of life and sexuality. J Clin Nurs 2001;10:221–9.

[54] Reynolds KE, Magnan MA. Nursing attitudes and beliefs toward human sexuality. Clin Nurse Spec 2005;19(5):255–9.

[55] Althof S, Rosen R, Rogatis L, et al. Outcome measurement in female sexual dysfunction clinical trials. J Sex Marital Ther 2005;31(2):153–66.

ELSEVIER
SAUNDERS

Nurs Clin N Am 42 (2007) 531–554

NURSING
CLINICS
OF NORTH AMERICA

Sexuality in Women with Cancer

Margaret Barton-Burke, PhD, RN[a,b,c,]*,
Carolyn J. Gustason, RN, BSN, OCN[d]

[a]*University of Massachusetts Amherst, Amherst, MA, USA*
[b]*The Phyllis F. Cantor Center, Dana-Farber Cancer Institute, Boston, Massachusetts, USA*
[c]*Yvonne L. Munn Center for Nursing Research, The Institute for Patient Care,
Massachusetts General Hospital, Boston, Massachusetts, USA*
[d]*Cancer Center, Clinical Research Office, University of Massachusetts Medical School,
Worcester, MA, USA*

"The truth of it is that I don't feel like a woman most of the time. I wear my hair long on purpose... [as she is crying] I don't cry much about this anymore... but I wear my hair long because this is all I have left that makes me female. I don't have boobs and ovaries and I don't have sex in my life and so I can grow my hair."
...Suzanne, 42 years old, diagnosed with breast cancer at 36 years of age from Barton-Burke, 2002 [1].

The American Cancer Society (ACS) estimates that there will be 678,060 new cases of cancer diagnosed in women in 2007. The majority (52%) of these cancers are expected to be diagnosed in the breast (26%), the lung (15%), and the colon and rectum (11%); the remainder (48%) of the cancers found in women account for tumors of the uterus and ovary, kidney, thyroid, and melanoma as well as leukemias and lymphomas [2]. The number of women surviving cancer is on the rise with reports from the Institute of Medicine (IOM) and other agencies indicating that between 8.9 and 10 million Americans have a history of cancer and that the number of cancer survivors is expected to continue to rise as the population ages [3]. These survival statistics highlight the success of screening and early detection and newer, more aggressive and increasingly complex treatment regimens combining radiation therapy, surgery, chemotherapy, and targeted therapies to cure or at least control many forms of cancer.

Based on these survival statistics, many women with cancer diagnosed in the last decade are either in active treatment or are classified as cured but

* Corresponding author.
E-mail address: bartonburkem@prodigy.net (M. Barton-Burke).

0029-6465/07/$ - see front matter © 2007 Elsevier Inc. All rights reserved.
doi:10.1016/j.cnur.2007.08.001
nursing.theclinics.com

living with the long-term effects of the disease or its treatment. Cancer treatments and their side effects often leave women with permanent and disabling sequelae; these sequelae are often dependent on the cancer diagnosed, the organ(s) involved, the treatment modalities used, and pre-existing comorbid diseases. Additionally, the cancer or the treatment sequelae may not be evident until years after treatment is complete. The sexuality of women with cancer is one sequelae of cancer that requires attention as a diagnosis, treatment, and survivor phenomenon. The purpose of this article is to review the evidence that is available to date about sexuality in women with cancer.

Sexuality and cancer

Sexuality is a comprehensive term encompassing an integration of physical, psychological, and social dimensions of sexual beings in ways that are positively enriching and enhance personality, communication, and love. Sexuality involves more than the sex act and reproduction; it encompasses who and what we are as a man or woman, how we get that way, how we feel about it, and how we deal with each other about it. Sexuality consists of sexual drive, sexual activities, intimacy and physical closeness, expressions of maleness and femaleness, and gender identity. Influencing factors include societal norms, religious background and culture, and health and illness. Research findings suggest that from 20% to 90% of cancer patients experience sexual problems either as a consequence of the disease itself or as a side effect of treatment [4,5].

Review of the literature was performed using the Pub Med and Cumulative Index to Nursing and Allied Health Literature (CINAHL) databases. Search terms included "libido and female cancer survivors," "quality of life and sexuality," "elderly female cancer survivors and sexual dysfunction," "sexual functioning and female and cancer," "female cancer survivors and sexuality," and "libido and menopausal female cancer survivors." Table 1 summarizes the research done within the last 12 years on the topic of sexuality in women with cancer. Table 2 is a summary of the literature by type of cancer and the effects on sexuality, sexual function, fertility, partners, and the clinical implications.

Many cancers, such as breast, ovarian, and uterine, have a direct effect on women's sex organs, and much is written about the sexuality of women with these cancers [6–20]. The majority of study results come from a population of women with breast cancer. This research has methodologic and design concerns because most studies are descriptive with sample limitations such as varying sample sizes. The results of these studies continue to confirm that women who are diagnosed with, treated for, and living with cancer experience problems with their sexuality. Gaps exist in areas of research such as late effects with long-term survivors, impact on older women, and underrepresentation of minorities, medically underserved, poor, and hard to reach populations.

The exception to the gaps are studies by Wilmoth [21–27], whose writings have added depth and breadth to our understanding of the types and kinds of sexual concerns women have after being treated for cancer. Her instrument, the Wilmoth Sexual Behavior Questionnaire–Female, is a valid and reliable tool that is useful when measuring female sexuality [28]. Wilmoth and Sanders [29], Ashing-Giwa and colleagues [30], Taylor and colleagues [31], and Adams and colleagues [32] found that changes in sexual relationships after a diagnosis of and treatment for cancer were a cultural construction as well. Additionally Barton-Burke [33] in her current qualitative, descriptive study found that sexuality was not discussed with unmarried black women and that the language that black women might use to discuss sexuality may not be the same as that spoken by the health care providers.

The following quotes illustrate these findings:

"...nobody asked me about my sexuality or whatever and it's not about how's your sex life? Being single, I think what's important for health care providers to ask is, I guess the cancer was always the focus. (Paula, 10-year survivor)

"...how attractive would I be to a man without my breasts and right now? I think about pain versus a man, pain versus a man, no pain, no man.... I was intimate with someone that I felt comfortable with just to see if I would get wet after the hysterectomy and that was over two months after I had it and I did and I was pleased and that was the end of that..." (Victoria, 3-year survivor)

"...it's talked about after mastectomy and we didn't talk on it but I should have talked on it because I'm dealing with this, the loss of my nipple and a lot of women I'm sure enjoyed the sensation sexually of having their nipple, and now it's gone and before I had this surgery when they suggested me to have this surgery, they never told me that I would have no nipple. Well yes they said you can get one but they didn't tell me that there was no feeling and there would be no feeling in my abdomen and it would itch and... yes, that bothers me. They didn't tell me that and I told the doctor that I was upset. I told the doctor because they're going to hire another plastic surgeon, and I was like well I hope they tell the people the truth because when they offered me this surgery they were like oh come on and you'll have this nice flat stomach but they never told me the side effects, the other stuff. They didn't tell me." (Missy, 3-year survivor)

Finally, little is known about women and their families including the impact of cancer on female children and their sexual and reproductive development or the multicultural issues facing long-term survivors and the long-term effects of less frequently studied cancers, and there are few studies beyond 5 years [34].

As mentioned earlier, the majority of research on women and sexuality has been conducted with women who were being treated for breast cancer. Research findings focus on symptom complaints related to treatment side effects from radiation and chemotherapy and address sexual dysfunction in women after diagnosis and treatment [6,7,10,12,13,19,35–37]. These

Table 1
Research conducted about sexuality in women with cancer

Disease site	Reference	Population	Research findings
Breast	Avis et al [6]	204 women ≤50 years of age.	Women who received chemotherapy reported more sexual difficulties than did younger women. Women experienced more menopausal-type symptoms than age-matched peers.
	Brandberg et al [7]	408 Scandinavian women.	Women who had mastectomies reported less sexual interest.
	Burwell et al [8]	209 women from New England area.	Sexual functioning impaired during chemotherapy treatment and for at least 42 weeks after the end of chemotherapy treatment. Sexual dysfunction decreases over time.
	Dorval et al [9]	124 breast cancer survivors compared with 262 controls.	Lesser degree of satisfaction with sex lives reported by breast cancer survivors than women in control group.
	Ganz et al [10]	558 women in transitional period between end of treatment and start of survivorship.	Chemotherapy was associated with more sexual dysfunction. Women who believed the cancer diagnosis had a negative effect on their life reported a decrease in vaginal lubrication and more sexual difficulties.
	Ganz et al [38]	76 postmenopausal women.	Development and testing of "Comprehensive Menopausal Assessment" had a statistically significant positive increase in levels of sexual functioning in experimental group.
	Ganz et al [11]	1134 women from 2 large metropolitan cities.	Identified key predictors of sexual health to be presence or absence of vaginal dryness, emotional well-being, body image, quality of intimate relationship, and whether the partner had sexual problems.
	Ganz et al [12]	864 women.	Chemotherapy treatment contributes to poorer sexual functioning. Tamoxifen did not have a significant impact on sexual functioning in women 50 years of age and older.
	Geiger et al [57]	519 women who did/did not undergo a contralateral prophylactic mastectomy.	Less contentment associated with dissatisfaction with sex life; 40.9% reported satisfaction with sex life, whereas 59.1% reported dissatisfaction.

Henson [13]	Literature review.	Chemotherapy associated with more sexual dysfunction. Breast conservation therapy has not led to a demonstrated enhancement in sexual functioning among breast cancer survivors.
Knobf [46]	27 white women in late 30s to early 40s received adjuvant chemotherapy.	Most women experienced menopausal symptoms. The meaning a woman placed on her breast cancer affected her entire experience and shaped her decision-making process.
Kornblith et al [14]	153 women.	Approximately one third of participants reported sexual problems that they attributed to their cancer experience.
Shultz et al [15]	291 women.	Majority of women rated painful sexual intercourse as a problem; however, this did not appear to influence how the participants perceived cancers' effects on their overall health.
Speer et al [16]	55 women.	The amount of relationship dysfunction between woman and partner was variable related to sexual functioning.
Takahashi and Kai [17]	21 Japanese women.	Most experienced sexual changes after treatment for cancer. Several women experienced decreased sexual activity were not disturbed by that change.
Wilmoth and Townsend [35]	165 women.	Minimal alcohol use, absence of chemotherapy and absence of tamoxifen was found to have a significantly positive effect on sexuality.
Wilmoth and Ross [21]	105 women.	Physical and psychosocial changes caused by cancer and treatment includes changes in perception of one's "femaleness."
Wilmoth and Botchway [23]	Patients with breast and gynecologic cancers.	Review that provided information regarding cancer treatment-related side effects in a clear and easily understandable format.
Wilmoth [25]	18 white women.	Identified the core concept of the altered sexual self. Detailed the psychological tasks that must be completed before the woman can progress to an integrated altered sexual self.
Wilmoth and Sanders [29]	24 African-American women.	A menopausal theme was identified during focus groups with African-American women. This theme included changes in their sexual relationships including a decrease in the level of their sexual desire. The changes were felt to have a negative effect on their relationship with their partners. Culturally based discomfort in speaking of sexuality in a group setting was noted. Women were open to group educational activities surrounding sexuality issues from nursing staff.

(continued on next page)

Table 1 (*continued*)

Disease site	Reference	Population	Research findings
	Wyatt et al [51]	147 women from two large metropolitan cities; 51 women reported history of childhood sexual abuse, 11 women reported a history of penetrative childhood sexual abuse.	A history of penetrative childhood sexual abuse was associated with greater emotional distress.
Colorectal	Mannaerts et al [39]	79 rectal cancer survivors; approximately 30 women.	Sexual dysfunction associated with nerve injury secondary to the oncologic surgery.
	Marijnen et al [40]	990 rectal cancer survivors; 365 women.	While decreased sexual activity did not correlate with a decreased quality of life, patients who were no longer sexually active responded with a lower perceived sense of overall health. Preoperative radiation therapy was related to increased sexual dysfunction as compared with postoperative radiation therapy.
Gynecologic	Ashing-Giwa et al [30]	51 women from differing cultures: African-Americans, Latinas, Asian Americans and white women. The African-American women carried a diagnosis of cervical dysplasia.	Qualitative research study using focus group format to discover how diagnosis of cervical dysplasia or cancer affected women of different cultures. Sexual and relationship difficulties were identified. Women reported both physical and culturally influenced psychosocial issues associated with respective illness and resulting treatments.
	Carmack Taylor et al [18]	232 women.	Greater physical and psychosocial morbidities were positively associated with greater sexual dysfunction. Relationship status, age, psychosocial health and lack of current chemotherapeutic treatment were found to be predictive of satisfactory sexual functioning.

	Frumovitz et al [19]	74 cervical cancer survivors; 40 women as controls.	Radiation therapy was associated with greater menopausal symptoms, greater sexual dysfunction, and poorer reported global well-being. Sexual dysfunction continued up to 5 or more years after treatment with radiation therapy. Conversely, patients who had surgical treatment reported decreasing morbidity as more time passed since surgery and reported a quality of life comparable to the controls.
	Lockwood-Rayermann [42]	Ovarian cancer survivors.	Marriage was associated with better physical health and sexual functioning. Sexual dysfunction is multifactorial and can be related to biophysical and psychosocial factors. In addition may be related to side effects of symptom management.
	Roos et al [20]	62 women, most with gynecologic cancers, 13 with bladder cancer.	Pelvic exenteration led to more sexual dysfunction. Younger women and more extensive surgery were variables associated with increased sexual dysfunction. Women who had reconstructive surgery such as a neovagina reported a higher self-esteem.
	Stewart et al [36]	200 women.	Three quarters of respondents rated their sex lives as adequate or poor. When asked to rate their sense of loss surrounding these issues, less than 100 women reported a moderate to severe sense of loss. Sense of loss surrounding fertility and sexuality differed by age of woman, with an increased sense of loss reported by younger partnered women. The treatment modality of radiation therapy was associated with sexual dysfunction. Over one half of the women reported continuing pain they associated with their cancer therapy.
Kidney	Anastasiadis et al [37]	84 renal cell cancer survivors; 42 of whom were women.	Women identified treatment variables, ie, chemotherapy, immunotherapy, and radiation therapy, as etiologies behind sexual dysfunction. Women with renal cancer reported sexual functioning of poorer quality than similarly aged women with breast cancer.

(continued on next page)

Table 1 (*continued*)

Disease site	Reference	Population	Research findings
General	Barton-Burke [5]		Table detailing changes in patient and partner's sexuality and fertility as a function of primary and secondary effects of cancer treatment and suggested interventions.
			Libido as a portion of one's sexuality.
	Barton et al [50]		Alterations in sexuality secondary to different but often overlapping psychosocial and physical etiologies.
	Katz [59]		Patients need information throughout the stages of cancer survivorship regarding changes that may occur because of the cancer or the treatment of cancer.
	Krebs [71]		Multiple biophysical and psychosocial changes secondary to cancer treatments.
	Pelusi [34]		Notes gaps in knowledge:
			Lack of evidence-based nursing interventions for cancer survivors and sexual dysfunction.
			Lack of research on cancer and sexuality as lived by the gay and lesbian community as well as those not in partnered relationships.
	Shell [41]		Comprehensive review of nursing interventions for sexual dysfunction in the cancer patient.
			Highlights the lack of evidence-based nursing interventions for sexual dysfunction in the cancer patient.
			Direct and indirect effects of cancer and treatments.

Shell [62]	Primary and secondary effects of cancer treatment.
	Gay and lesbian couples who have not disclosed their sexuality to their family, friends, and health care providers are at risk for isolation.
	Giving the patient and partner permission to experiment sexually as a nursing intervention.
Shell [64]	Older patients continue to be sexual beings.
	Assessment of the older patient should include developmental tasks as well as physical functioning.
	Discrete attention should be given to the privacy needs of the elderly resident residing in long-term care facilities.
Wilmoth [22]	The best treatment for sexual dysfunction in the cancer patient is early assessment.
	Assessments should begin broad and become problem focused dependent upon difficulties identified during the assessment phase.
Wilmoth et al [27]	Offers a literature review of the concept of symptom clusters in breast cancer survivors; specific symptoms explored are fatigue, weight gain, and altered sexuality.
	Biophysical and psychosocial etiologies of targeted symptoms explored with proposed interventions.

Table 2
Effects of cancer on sexuality, sexual function, fertility, partners, and clinical implications

Site	Dysfunction: physical	Dysfunction: psychological	Effect on fertility	Impact on partner	Comments	Implications for clinical practice
Breast Cancer						
Breast	The absence of foreplay using nipple stimulation for arousal may cause some difficulties.	Usually	Dependent on treatment used and age of women.	Usually	If oophorectomy and hormonal manipulations are used, can affect all aspects of sexuality.	Chemotherapeutic agents may cause ovarian failure with hot flashes and vaginal dryness. Poly-glycol-based, water-soluble vaginal lubricants should be used. Mastectomy: prosthesis and lingerie may conceal surgical site. Alternative positions for intercourse may be suggested to keep breast or scar out of sight, such as vaginal penetration from a side lying position or vaginal penetration from behind. To prevent unrealistic expectations after breast reconstruction, a drawing or photograph of how the new breast might look should be shown before the reconstruction. Cultural competency important when planning interventions.
Colon Cancer						
Colon/ Rectum	Usually; nerve damage may negatively affect sensation.	Usually; especially with formation of an ostomy.	None; except with XRT and chemotherapy.	Sometimes.	Women sometimes have a hysterectomy with the operative procedure. With ostomies and external collection devices, specific suggestions about emptying appliances before engaging in sex can relieve anxiety about leaksand odors.	Anterior resection is a surgical procedure with better sexual outcomes than abdominoperineal resection. Women report more positive sexual outcomes than men regardless of the surgical procedure. Dyspareunia may be present. Reports of perineal pain or phantom rectal pain.

Gynecologic Cancers

Cervix					
Treatment of in situ with cone biopsy will not cause dysfunction. Radical hysterectomy will shorten vagina 1/3 to 1/2; may be appreciable but usually not.	Sometimes.	No, with cone biopsy for in situ stages; yes, with hysterectomy and/or XRT.	Sometimes partner may feel that one can "catch" cancer or be affected by its treatment, especially XRT.	XRT to pelvis causes thickening of vagina and may cause stenosis or fistula formation and dyspareunia.	Deep pelvic thrusts may be painful; sexual positions may have to be modified to avoid discomfort, eg, woman on top, side lying position, creative use of pillows. Poly-glycol-based or water-soluble lubricants on a woman's thighs, which are then adducted during intercourse, can create the sensation of a deep vagina. Alternative position: vaginal penetration from behind between closely adducted thighs. Vaginal dilators used several times a week (three times is recommended) keeps vagina from stenosing. An alternative to using a vaginal dilator is to have intercourse a few times per week. Should be done for the remainder of her life. Poly-glycol-based, water-soluble lubricants recommended

(continued on next page)

Table 2 (*continued*)

Site	Dysfunction: physical	Dysfunction: psychological	Effect on fertility	Impact on partner	Comments	Implications for clinical practice
Uterus	Total abdominal hysterectomy with pelvic node dissection usually causes no dysfunction. XRT to pelvis causes thickening of the vagina if included in XRT fields.	Sometimes.	Yes, with either XRT or surgery.	Sometimes	Because of lack of literature on female sexual response, it is difficult to determine differences between physical and psychological dysfunction.	Menopausal changes of sudden onset in previously asymptomatic women include vaginal dryness and hot flashes. Vaginal lubricants, polyglycol-based and water-soluble suggested.
Ovary	In premenopausal women, bilateral oophorectomy results in menopausal symptoms.	Sometimes.	Yes, except with cases of unilateral oophorectomy	Sometimes.	Dyspareunia can occur. Germ cell ovarian tumors usually occur in one ovary. An oophorectomy of affected ovary should maintain fertility by preserving the uterus and other ovary.	If premenopausal, treatment of menopausal changes including vaginal dryness and hot flashes. Vaginal lubrication recommended. Chemotherapy may cause alopecia, nausea, vomiting, and fatigue, minimizing desire for sexual intercourse.

Vulva	Simple vulvectomy can result in introital stenosis. Radical vulvectomy includes removal of clitoris.	Usually.	No, patient often postmenopausal.	Usually.	Radical vulvectomy can cause a decrease in ROM of lower extremities.	Postoperative perineal numbness may impair arousal. After clitorectomy may be a decrease in or absence of orgasms. Need to relearn how to reach orgasm. Intercourse may be painful.
Other Cancers						
Bladder	Local–seldom: In women, cystectomy usually includes removal of bladder, urethra, uterus, and anterior vagina.	Usually.	Always with XRT.	Usually.	The development of continent urostomies has made the use of the ostomy bag unnecessary in many cases. Wearing a cummerbund, decorative stoma covering, or underwear with a crotch cut out may help.	In Women: there is limited research. Bladder cancer in women has similar sequelae to gynecologic cancers receiving an anterior pelvic exenteration with a narrow vagina. Dyspareunia resulting from vaginal tightness and lack of lubrication.
Hodgkin's lymphoma/ non-Hodgkin's lymphoma	The disease process and effects of therapy may decrease sexual drive and ability.	Sometimes.	Yes, with XRT to pelvis without shielding of gonads; chemotherapy may decrease ova maturation.	Usually.	Patients on chemotherapy alone should be using some form of contraception. The effects of chemotherapy on ova maturation is not totally understood. Extensive fatigue often diminishes sex drive and function.	Most frequent sequelae include poor body image, decreased sexual drive, and satisfaction. Further research is needed to determine multiple variables and their influence on sexuality in Hodgkin's lymphoma/non-Hodgkin's lymphoma survivors.

(continued on next page)

Table 2 (continued)

Site	Dysfunction: physical	Dysfunction: psychological	Effect on fertility	Impact on partner	Comments	Implications for clinical practice
Leukemia	The disease process and associated blood counts with chemotherapy may affect ability to participate in sexual activity.	Sometimes.	Chemotherapy affects ova maturation, but they may rebound after cessation of treatment.	Usually.	Patients on chemotherapy alone should be using some form of contraception. The effects of chemotherapy on ova maturation is not totally understood. Extensive fatigue often diminishes sex drive and function.	Most frequent sequelae include poor body image, decreased sexual drive, and satisfaction. Further research is needed to determine multiple variables and their influence on sexuality in leukemia survivors.

Chemotherapy, radiation, and analgesics all are associated with generalized feelings of malaise. This can have a profound effect on feelings of self-image, self-worth, sexuality, and libido. All these factors should be taken into consideration when assessing the sexual needs and/or problems of cancer patients and their families.

Abbreviations: XRT, radiation therapy; ROM, range of motion.

Data from Refs. [3,22,45,46] and Ganz PA, Litwin MS, Meyerowitz BE. Sexual problems. In: DeVita VT, Hellman S, Rosenberg SA, editors. Cancer: principles & practice of oncology (Books @ Ovid, Section 56.3). Philadelphia: Lippincott Williams & Wilkins; 2001; Halfin V, Morgantaler A, Barton Burke M, Goldstein I. Sexuality and cancer. In: Osteen R, editor. Cancer manual. Framingham (MA): American Cancer Society; 1996; Lamb ML, Woods NF. Sexuality and the cancer patient. Cancer Nursing 1981;4:138–9; American Cancer Society. (Sexuality and cancer for the woman who has cancer and her partner. Atlanta (GA): American Cancer Society; 2004; and Young-McCaughan S. Sexual functioning in women with breast cancer after treatment with adjuvant therapy. Cancer Nursing 1996;19(4):308–9.

reports offer evidence that is focused narrowly with conflicting results [9,15,16,38] including the fact that sexual dysfunction decreases over time [8].

We found no articles related to lung cancer, the second most prevalent cancer for women and sexuality per se. Later we discuss the symptom of dyspnea as a contributor to the sexual dysfunction in women with cancer. Our search for evidence-based research on the third most prevalent cancer diagnosed in women, colorectal cancer, yields few articles on the subject [39,40]. Findings from this literature suggest that there is a relationship between surgery and radiation therapy and sexual dysfunction in women undergoing treatment for this type of cancer. The evidence of research-based interventions and practices are almost nonexistent, yet there is evidence of expert opinion available to readers [41].

According the ACS, gynecologic cancers are not as prevalent as the other three types of cancer in women, yet there is a growing body of research on women with ovarian, cervical, and other cancers including renal cancers and cancer of the urinary bladder. This literature is fraught with small samples and studies that continue to be descriptive. These studies report that there are sexual sequelae to diagnosis and treatment, but intervention studies were not found in the literature reviewed for this article. Regardless of the cancer incidence, when cancer is diagnosed in female sex organs, these organs become a target for research investigation. The research reports that women with gynecologic cancers have symptoms, such as early menopause and dyspareunia, resulting from treatment [18–20,28,36,37,42,43].

Other cancers such as leukemia and lymphoma have a secondary effect on women and their sexuality by the quantity and quality of treatment side effects and from the enduring nature of those side effects. Although some research has been completed regarding the side effects of bone marrow transplants on the quality of life for men and women survivors, the samples were small and contained even smaller numbers of women. Participant responses were analyzed as part of a larger more heterogeneous age or symptom group and therefore had limited usefulness for application in this patient population [44].

Sexuality and cancer treatments

The treatments involved with any given cancer have the potential to alter sexual function. Surgery, chemotherapy, radiation, and biotherapy are known to contribute to sexual dysfunction in a variety of direct and indirect ways. The use of targeted therapies has not been in existence long enough, and there have been no studies available in the literature that suggest that these therapies are or are not implicated in the sexuality of women with cancer. Women identify surgery and chemotherapy as etiologies responsible for sexual dysfunction and report poorer sexual functioning than similarly aged women with breast cancer [37]. Sexuality for women with cancer is complicated by variables such as the type of cancer, the type of treatment used, the psychological changes in body image and social role, along with consequent distraction or preoccupation with bodily functions complicates. Fig. 1 is a simple model that highlights the impact of cancer and the treatments for cancer identifying the manifold effects that various cancer and its treatments have on sexuality in women with cancer.

Surgery affects sexual function when the tumor involves the sex or reproductive organs requiring surgical procedures such as mastectomy, vaginectomy, hysterectomy, or ostomy or when the surgical intervention affects function. Studies have found that sexual dysfunction was associated with nerve damage after surgery [39] and with preoperative radiation [40] for colon cancer. Postsurgical pain from mastectomy, thoracotomy, head and neck surgery, or amputation is well established in the literature and is treated symptomatically [45].

Radiation therapy directly and indirectly affects one's sexuality by virtue of tissue and organ damage. For example, brachytherapy for the treatment of cervical cancer is known to cause vaginal stenosis. Additionally, radiation therapy to the abdomen can directly affect the gastrointestinal mucosa, resulting in diarrhea, which can indirectly affect sexual function [5].

Chemotherapeutic agents have side effects that can either directly or indirectly affect sexuality and sexual function. Cytotoxic chemotherapy can affect female fertility as well as function. Direct damage to the ovaries may induce a premature menopause. Other side effects of chemotherapy include the masculinizing or feminizing effects of treatment, which can alter

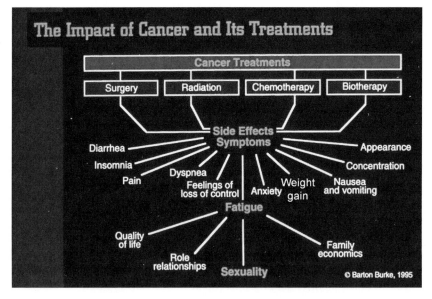

Fig. 1. The impact of cancer and its treatments (*Courtesy of* Margaret Barton-Burke, PhD, RN, Boston, MA).

one's libido [15,21,46,47]. Many agents affect sexuality indirectly because of their side-effect profile; examples include nausea, vomiting, and alopecia.

Biotherapy directly causes severe fatigue that affects activities of daily life and quality of that life [48], and although there is no literature about sexuality and sexual functioning for patients receiving these therapies, we can extrapolate our knowledge about fatigue for women with cancer.

Cancer-related fatigue is the most frequent complaint of cancer survivors with few studies on its impact on sexuality. Recent findings about symptom clustering in women with cancer suggest that fatigue, sleep disturbances, pain, anxiety, and depression are symptoms that cluster [49]. Once again, findings could be extrapolated about this symptom cluster because studies found significant relationships between cancer-related fatigue and sleep disturbances [49]. Few findings suggest the actual impact of these symptoms on sexuality in women diagnosed with, treated for, and living with the sequelae of cancer. Further research on the prevalence of this symptom cluster and its effect on the sexuality of women with cancer can inform clinical practice.

Research about sexuality in women with cancer who have received treatment with chemotherapy or radiation therapy has focused on pain, fatigue, weight gain, nausea and vomiting, and alopecia, any or all of which can make a woman feel less sexually attractive [25]. Treatment sequelae may contribute to psychological reactions such as depression that may be associated with a decrease in sexual drive. Medications may affect sexual functioning or responsiveness [50,51].

Frequently women who survive cancer experience long-term changes such as impaired vital organ dysfunction, hormonal changes resulting in infertility and altered sexual function, cognitive changes, ongoing fatigue, depression, anxiety, family distress, and economic challenges that can all contribute to a woman's sexuality and sexual function [25,30,46,47]. In particular, premature menopause results in changes related to natural hormone loss and androgen deprivation therapy. Women who become menopausal have between 63% and 96% bone loss within 1 year and the American Society of Clinical Oncology (ASCO) has developed screening guidelines and treatment recommendations for breast cancer survivors [52].

Cancer treatments affect the cardiac and pulmonary organ systems incurring symptoms such as tachycardia, nonproductive cough, and electrocardiograph (EKG) changes. If Adriamycin or bleomycin or other cardio- or pulmono-toxic treatments were used during therapy, symptoms such as dyspnea may affect the energy that is necessary for sexual activity [53].

Informed consent for cancer treatment including information about the reproductive issues must be given before the start of therapy, and such information should include genetic alterations and the possibility of assisted reproduction options. Fertility and infertility options, such as cryopreservation of oocytes, embryo, and ovarian tissue, must be offered to cancer patients before starting treatment [5,46].

Other ongoing problems that can affect sexuality and sexual function include pain and neuropathy. Pain and neuropathy related to surgery, radiation therapy, and chemotherapy are treated with a variety of agents, such as anticonvulsants, tricyclic antidepressants, opioids, glutamine, glutathione, amifostine, and vitamin E. Additionally, exercise interventions and nutritional supplements are all in various states of clinical trials [45].

Finally, the effect of treatments on sexuality may result from the assault on one's body image by the diagnosis, treatment, or treatment sequelae. There is some research to support the fact that there may be a discrepancy between a woman's perception of her body image and the reality of the actual body image [34,54]. As a result of early detection and better treatment, cancer has progressed from an exclusively fatal disease to a chronic illness [13,55,56], making quality-of-life issues such as sexuality increasingly important as patients move from a time of cancer diagnosis into survivorship [5,19,21,27,33,57–59].

The older woman with cancer and her sexuality

Cancer is a disease of aging. Findings that the number of cancer patients over the age of 60 will double in the next 30 years [55] combined with census data indicating a 60% increase in the number of women over the age of 64 by the year 2040 suggest the need for a better understanding of the older women with cancer [60,61]. One area lacking research and evidence-based practice is the older woman with cancer and her sexuality.

Most people, including older women, are sexual beings throughout much of their lives, and this interest does not end at menopause or at her sixty-fifth birthday. Many women remain sexually active as they age [62–64]. Age-related changes that occur that may influence the older woman's sexuality include (1) an aging sometimes ill body, (2) the loss of a long term partner, (3) changes in a partner's ability or desire to function in a sexual manner, and (4) changes in living arrangements. Expert knowledge about the impact of cancer treatment on the older woman's sexuality becomes even more important as the population of women with cancer ages [21].

Little is written about evidence-based practices that address older women with cancer and sexual functioning. Most articles include small samples of women over the age of 65, but when the sample included women 65 years of age and older, participant responses were analyzed as part of a larger more heterogeneous age group, thus limiting the usefulness of the findings to a population of older women with cancer. Similarly, reports addressing the specific population of the older cancer survivor did not include information about women's sexuality within the scope of their work [56,65–67]. When found, interventions were based on expert opinions and mirrored those used with younger women [25,30,37,44,64].

There is a paucity of evidence-based nursing research on the needs of the older women with cancer in general and their sexuality in particular. There is a need for research about the effects of cancer treatments in older women, the responses—both physical and psychological—to these treatments, and evidenced-based care and research-based interventions in this population [34,56,66–68]. Additionally, areas of research must include the meaning of sexuality to elderly women who have survived cancer, similarities and differences that may exist between different socioeconomic groups, different ethnic and racial groups, and differences that may or may not exist depending on one's sexual orientation, one's religious identity, or one's geographic location. The conduct, analysis and dissemination of knowledge gained from this type of investigation will assist nurses in providing evidence-based care to this growing segment of society [69].

There is an age, gender, and marital status bias that pervades the manner in which sexual assessments are conducted. There is a presumption that the person with cancer has a sexual partner who is a member of the opposite sex. Single individuals may be highly active sexually and may be more concerned about changes in sexuality and sexual function than their married or partnered counterparts. Knowing patients' sexual orientation is not as important as assessing for changes in patients' usual sexual practices. Nonjudgmental inquiries about sexual behavior can help minimize the bias of an assessment and can make the patient feel more comfortable revealing information about her sexuality.

Implications for nursing practice

The impetus in health care today for evidenced-based practice has provided us with the drive to determine "the evidence." Nurses are seeking evidenced-based practice guidelines for interventions based on research that is organized by the quantity and strength of the research findings. The guidelines based on such research recommendations range from *recommended for practice* in which interventions are supported by strong evidence to *effectiveness unlikely* in which research produced no effect or were from poorly controlled or uncontrolled trials. The findings from methodologically rigorous studies are expected to increase our knowledge of the burden of illness, yield key information regarding follow-up care, and facilitate the development of best practice guidelines [37,70].

National organizations, such as the National Comprehensive Cancer Network (NCCN) and the Oncology Nursing Society (ONS), are developing evidence-based practice guidelines for many cancers or cancer-related conditions such as fatigue. A search of a variety of websites finds no practice guidelines related to sexuality and cancer. Some national organizations have resources for sexuality for women with cancer. The American Cancer Society (ACS), *http://www.cancer.org*, has the booklet entitled, *Sexuality & Cancer—For The Woman With Cancer*. While the National Cancer Institute (NCI), *http://www.cancer.gov/cancerinfo/pdq/supportivecare/sexuality/patient*, has documents available in their Physician Query Database (PDQ). The titles available are *Sexuality and Reproductive Issues (PQD) (Patient)* and *Sexuality and Reproductive Issues (PQD) (Health Professionals)*. There are Spanish language versions of these documents that can be found at *http://www.cancer.gov/espanol/pdq/cuidados-medicos-apoyo/sexualidad/Health Professional*. The NCI has the topic of sexuality embedded in other publications as well: *Taking Time* and program publications like the *Facing Forward Series: Life after Cancer Treatment* can be found at *http://www.cancer.gov/cancerinfo/life-after-treatment*.

More work is needed to develop the scientific basis for practice interventions for sexuality in women with cancer. Intervention studies are necessary. but how they would be developed, operationalized, and conducted in an ethical manner is one possible reason for the dearth of this research in the literature. Empirically we know that there are barriers to interventions surrounding sexuality in women with cancer that stem from implicit assumptions about sexuality on the part of both the patient and the provider. The topic of sexuality may not be discussed with the patient by the provider; conversely, the patient may not raise the topic.

Regardless of who initiates it, communication is a key element for both the patient and the provider. A willingness to discuss sexual history and to ask clear questions about sexual functioning before and after diagnosis and treatment are ways to open or encourage a dialog about sexuality. Incorporating basic questions into the review of systems can introduce the topic and serve as a starting point for more detailed inquiry. Patients report that they would like to discuss sexual issues with their health care provider but are reluctant to do so [71]. It is recommended that discussion of potential sexual problems begin at the time of diagnosis, letting patients know they have permission to discuss the subject whenever necessary [71]. The sexual partner plays a pivotal role, and whenever possible partners should be included in these discussions.

A history of cancer, changes in appearance and body image, and uncertainty about fertility can contribute to a cancer survivor's concern about sexual function. Fertility is an important topic to discuss especially during the discussion of treatment options. Strategies to conserve fertility often are used, but they are highly dependent on the type of cancer, the treatment, and geographic availability. Approaches to preserve ovarian tissue with subsequent reimplantation are options for women of childbearing age. Specific suggestions with information may help patients understand their options and help them make informed treatment decisions.

Issues related to sexuality and sexual function can arise at any time, and it is important to note that problems with sexual function may not be a result of the diagnosis and treatments alone. Pre-existing problems may be exacerbated by the diagnosis of cancer. An understanding of the disease, organs involved, treatment used, and long-term effects, allows the nurse to inform patients about what to expect from their experience with cancer.

Pending the completion of scientifically sound evidenced-based research, the nurse has the option of using, with caution, interventions as noted in the literature. Such interventions include early assessment of sexual functioning, avoidance of heterosexism, assisting the patient in the redefinition of intimacy [64], patient education surrounding normal age-related changes [64], and the effects cancer treatment (ie, surgery, radiation therapy, hormonal therapy, targeted therapy, and chemotherapy) may have on their body.

Summary

The purpose of this report was to review the evidence that is available to date about sexuality in women with cancer. There is a vast amount of information on this topic, much of which is not evidenced based. However, there is an expanding body of scientific evidence published by a small number of researchers that is shedding light on our knowledge about sexuality in women with cancer. Much of this research describes and measures the phenomenon. There are gaps in the research, making the interventions that are used more expert opinion rather than science. There is a need for research about effective interventions, and there is a need to educate nurses to help change practice through communication about a topic that makes both the patient and the nurse uncomfortable. However, as patients are living longer after a diagnosis of cancer, nurses can be pivotal in changing the status quo and begin to discuss sexuality in women with cancer just like we could discuss any other quality-of-life issue as it relates to cancer.

References

[1] Barton-Burke M. Breast cancer experiences: women's reflections years after diagnosis. Kingston (RI): University of Rhode Island, 2002.

[2] American Cancer Society. Cancer facts and figures 2007. Atlanta (GA): American Cancer Society; 2007.

[3] Hewitt M, Greenfield S, Stovall E, editors, and the Committee on Cancer Survivorship; improving care and quality of life, National Cancer Policy Board, institutes of medicine. From cancer patient to cancer survivor: LOST in transition. Washington (DC): National Academies Press; 2005.

[4] Andersen BL, Lamb MA. Sexuality and cancer. In: Murphy GP, Lawrence W, Lenhard RE, editors. American cancer society textbook for clinical oncology. 2nd edition. Atlanta (GA): American Cancer Society; 1995. p. 699–713.

[5] Barton-Burke M. Sexuality. In: Varricchio CG, editor. A cancer sourcebook for nurses. 8th edition. Sudbury (MA): Jones and Bartlett Publishers; 2004. p. 467–8.

[6] Avis NE, Crawford S, Manuel J. Psychosocial problems among younger women with breast cancer. Psycho-oncology 2004;13(July 2004):295–308.

[7] Brandberg Y, Michelson H, Nilsson B, et al. Quality of life in women with breast cancer during the first year after random assignment to adjuvant treatment with marrow-supported high-dose chemotherapy with cyclophosphamide, thiotepa, and carboplatin or tailored therapy with fluorouracil, epirubicin. J Clin Oncol 2003;21(19):3959–3664.

[8] Burwell SR, Case LD, Kaelin C, et al. Sexual problems in younger women after breast cancer surgery. J Clin Oncol 2006;24(18):2815–21.

[9] Dorval M, Maunsell E, Deschenes E, et al. Long-term quality of life after breast cancer: Comparison of 8-year survivors with population controls. J Clin Oncol 1998;16(2):487–94.

[10] Ganz PA, Kwan L, Stanton AL, et al. Quality of life at the end of primary treatment of breast cancer: First results from the moving beyond cancer randomized trial. Journal of the American Cancer Institute 2004;96(5):376–87.

[11] Ganz PA, Desmond KA, Belin TR, et al. Predictors of sexual health in women after a breast cancer diagnosis. J Clin Oncol 1999;17(8):2371–80.

[12] Ganz PA, Rowland JH, Desmond K, et al. Life after breast cancer: Understanding women's health-related quality of life and sexual functioning. J Clin Oncol 16(2):501–14.

[13] Henson HK. Breast cancer and sexuality. Sex Disabil 2002;20(4):261–75.

[14] Kornblith AB, Herdon JE II, Weiss RB, et al. Long-term adjustment of survivors of early-stage breast carcinoma, 20 years after adjuvant chemotherapy. Cancer 2003;98(4): 679–89.

[15] Shultz PN, Klein MJ, Beck ML, et al. Breast cancer: relationship between menopausal symptoms, physiologic health effects of cancer treatment and physical constraints on quality of life in long-term survivors. J Clin Nurs 2005;14:204–11.

[16] Speer JJ, Hillenberg B, Sugrue DP, et al. Study of sexual functioning determinants in breast cancer survivors. Breast J 2005;11(6):440–7.

[17] Takahashi M, Kai I. Sexuality after breast cancer treatment: Changes and coping strategies among Japanese survivors. Soc Sci Med 2005;61:1278–90.

[18] Carmack Taylor CL, Basen-Enquist K, Shinn E, et al. Predictors of sexual functioning in ovarian cancer patients. J Clin Oncol 2004;22(5):881–9.

[19] Frumovitz M, Sun CC, Shover LR, et al. Quality of life and sexual functioning in cervical cancer survivors. J Clin Oncol 2005;23(30):7428–36.

[20] Roos EJ, de Graff A, van Eijkeren MA, et al. Quality of life after pelvic exenteration. Gynecol Oncol 2004;93:610–4.

[21] Wilmoth MC, Ross JA. Women's perceptions breast cancer treatments and sexuality. Cancer Pract 1997;5(6):353–9.

[22] Wilmoth MC. Sexuality resources for cancer professionals and their patients. Cancer Pract 1998;6(6):346–8.

[23] Wilmoth MC, Botchway P. Psychosexual implications of breast and gynecologic cancer. Cancer Invest 1999;17(8):631–6.

[24] Wilmoth MC, Spinelli A. Sexual implications of gynecologic cancer treatments. J Obstet Gynecol Neonatal Nurs 2000;413–21.

[25] Wilmoth MC. The aftermath of breast cancer: an altered sexual self. Cancer Nurs 2001;24(4): 278–86.

[26] Wilmoth MC, Bruner DW. Integrating sexuality into cancer nursing practice. Oncology Nursing patient treatment and support 2002;9(1):1–14.

[27] Wilmoth MC, Coleman EA, Smith SC, et al. Fatigue, weight gain and altered sexuality in patients with breast cancer: exploration of a symptom cluster. Oncol Nurs Forum 2004; 31(6):1069–73.

[28] Wilmoth MC, Tingle LR. Development and psychometric testing of the Wilmoth sexual behaviors questionnaire- female. Can J Nurs Res 2001;32(4):135–51.

[29] Wilmoth MC, Sanders LD. Accept me for myself: African American Women's Issues after breast cancer. Oncol Nurs Forum 2001;28(5):875–9.

[30] Ashing-Giwa KT, Kagawa-Singer M, Padilla GV, et al. The impact of cervical cancer and dysplasia: a qualitative multiethnic study. Psycho-oncology 2004;13:709–28.

[31] Taylor KL, Lamdan RM, Siegel JE, et al. Treatment regimen, sexual attractiveness concerns and psychological adjustment among African American breast cancer patient. Psycho-oncology 2002;11:505–17.

[32] Adams J, DeJesus Y, Trujillio M, et al. Assessing sexual dimensions in Hispanic women: development of an instrument. Cancer Nurs 1997;20(4):251–9.

[33] Barton-Burke M. Breast cancer experiences: Black women's reflections years after diagnosis. Preliminary findings from American cancer Society Institutional Research Grant. Worcester (MA): University of Massachusetts Medical School, 2007.

[34] Pelusi J. Sexuality and body image: research on breast cancer survivors documents altered body image and sexuality. Am J Nurs 2006;106(3):32–8.

[35] Wilmoth MC, Townsend J. A comparison of the effects of lumpectomy versus mastectomy on sexual behaviors. Cancer Pract 1995;3(5):279–85.

[36] Stewart DJ, Wong MBBS, Duff S. What doesn't kill you makes you stronger: An ovarian cancer survivor survey. Gynecol Oncol 2001;83:537–42.

[37] Anastasiadis A, Davis AR, Sawczuk IS, et al. Quality of life aspects in kidney cancer patients: data from a national registry. Support Care Cancer 2003;11:700–6.

[38] Ganz PA, Greendale GA, Petersen L, et al. Managing menopausal symptoms in breast cancer survivors: Results of a randomized controlled trial. J Natl Cancer Inst 2000;92(13): 1054–64.

[39] Mannaerts GHH, Schjiven MP, Hendrikx A, et al. Urologic and sexual morbidity following multimodality treatment for locally advanced primary and locally recurrent rectal cancer. Eur J Surg Oncol 2001;27:265–72.

[40] Marijinen CAM, van de Valde CJH, Putter H, et al. Impact of short-term preoperative radiotherapy on health-related quality of life and sexual functioning in primary rectal cancer: a report of a multicenter randomized trial. J Clin Oncol 2005;23(9):1847–58.

[41] Shell JA. Evidence-based practice for symptom management in adults with cancer: sexual dysfunction. Oncol Nurs Forum 2002;29(1):53–66.

[42] Lockwood-Rayermann S. Survivorship issues in ovarian cancer. Oncology Nursing 2006; 33(3):553–62.

[43] Stead M. Sexual dysfunction after treatment for gynaecologic and breast malignancies. Curr Opin Obstet Gynecol 2003;15(1):57–61.

[44] Hayden RJ, Keogh F, Ni Conghaile M, et al. A single-centre assessment of long term quality-of-life status after sibling allogenic stem cell transplantation for chronic myeloid leukemia in first chronic phase. Bone Marrow Transplant 2004;34(6):545–56.

[45] Polomano RC, Sarrar JT. Pain and neuropathy in cancer survivors. Am J Nurs 2006;106(3): 39–47.

[46] Knobf MT. The menopausal symptom experience in young mid-life women with breast cancer. Cancer Nurs 2001;24(3):201–10.

[47] Knobf MT. Reproductive and hormonal sequelae of chemotherapy in women. Am J Nurs 2006;106(3):60–5.

[48] Quesada J, Talpaz M, Rios A, et al. Clinical toxicity of interferons in cancer patients: A review. J Clin Oncol 1986;4(2):234–43.

[49] Barton-Burke M. Cancer related fatigue and sleep disturbances. Am J Nurs 2006;106(3): 72–7.

[50] Barton D, Wilwerding M, Carpenter L, et al. Libido as part of sexuality in female cancer survivors. Oncol Nurs Forum 2004;31(3):599–607.

[51] Wyatt GE, Loeb TB, Desmond KA, et al. Does a history of childhood sexual abuse affect sexual outcomes in breast cancer survivors? J Clin Oncol 2005;23(6):1261–9.

[52] Hawkins R. Osteoporosis. Am J Nurs 2006;106(3):78–82.

[53] Camp-Sorrell D. Cardiorespiratory effects in cancer survivors. Am J Nurs 2006;106(3):55–9.

[54] Hordern A. Intimacy and sexuality for the woman with breast cancer. Cancer nursing 2000; 23(3):230–6.

[55] Edwards BK, Howe HL, Ries L, et al. Annual report to the nation on the status of cancer, 1973–1999, featuring implications of age and aging on U.S. cancer burden. Cancer 2002; 94(10):2766–92.

[56] Bourbonniere M, Van Cleave JH. Cancer care in nursing homes. Semin Oncol Nurs 2006; 22(1):51–7.

[57] Geiger AM, West CN, Nekhlyudov L, et al. Contentment with quality of life among breast cancer survivors with and without contralateral prophylactic mastectomy. J Clin Oncol 2006;24(9):1350–6.

[58] Ganz PA, Guadagnoli E, Landrum MB, et al. Breast cancer in older women: Quality of life and psychosocial adjustment in the 15 months after diagnosis. J Clin Oncol 2003;21(21): 4027–33.

[59] Katz A. The sounds of silence: sexuality information for cancer patients. J Clin Oncol 2005; 23(1):238–41.

[60] U.S. Census Bureau. 2004. U.S. Interim projections by age, sex, race, and Hispanic origin. Available at: http://www.census.gov/ipc/www/usinterimproj/Internet. Accessed March 18, 2004.

[61] Heidrich SM, Egan JJ, Hengudomsub P, et al. Symptoms, symptom beliefs, and quality of life of older breast cancer survivors: a comparative study. Oncol Nurs Forum 2006;33(2): 315–22.

[62] Shell JA. Do you like the things that life is showing you? The sensitive self-image of the person with cancer. Oncol Nurs Forum 1995;22(6):907–11.

[63] Shell JA, Smith CK. Sexuality and the older person with cancer. Oncol Nurs Forum 1994; 21(3):553–8.

[64] Shell JA. Sexuality care of the older adult with cancer. In: Cope DG, Reb AM, editors. Treatment and care of the older adult with cancer. Pittsburgh (PA): (Oncology Nursing Society); 2006. p. 439–64.

[65] Dendurluri N, Ershler WB. Aging biology and cancer. Semin Oncol 2004;31(2):137–48.

[66] Lichtman SM. Chemotherapy in the elderly. Semin Oncol 2004;31(2):160–74.

[67] Kagan SH. Gero-oncology nursing research. Oncol Nurs Forum 2004;31(2):293–9.

[68] Reiner A, LaCasse C. Symptom correlates in the gero-oncology population. Semin Oncol Nurs 2006;22(1):20–30.

[69] Cochran S, Mays V, Bowen D, et al. Cancer-related risk indicators and preventive screening behaviors among lesbians and bisexual women. Am J Public Health 2001;91(4):591–7.

[70] Best practices: a guide to clinical excellence in nursing care. Philadelphia: Lippincott, Williams and Wilkins; 2003.

[71] Krebs L. What should I say? Talking with patients about sexuality issues. Clin J Oncol Nurs 2006;10(3):313–5.

ELSEVIER
SAUNDERS

Nurs Clin N Am 42 (2007) 555–580

NURSING
CLINICS
OF NORTH AMERICA

The Sexual Impact of Cancer and Cancer Treatments in Men

Deborah Watkins Bruner, RN, PhD[a,b,*],
Tammy Calvano, MA[a]

[a]School of Nursing, University of Pennsylvania, 418 Curie Boulevard,
Philadelphia, PA 19104, USA
[b]Recruitment, Retention and Outreach Core Facility, Abramson Cancer Center,
University of Pennsylvania, 418 Curie Boulevard,
Philadelphia, PA 19104, USA

With the Food and Drug Administration (FDA) approval of sildenafil in 1998, the first oral medication demonstrating significant efficacy across a variety of erectile dysfunction (ED) etiologies, there has been a plethora of publications devoted to ED. Along with this has come an increased interest in the pathophysiology of ED among numerous diseases, including cancer. While this has served to move evidence-based therapy forward, there remain significant gaps in the literature regarding the multifaceted aspects of male sexuality beyond ED, including libido, sexual satisfaction, body image, and relationships. In addition, in the cancer literature to date, most of the research assessing the effectiveness of methods to improve ED following cancer therapy has focused on prostate cancer. There is a continuing need for the study of sexual function following therapy for other cancers affecting men, from testicular to lung and colon cancers, among others. This article presents an overview of the literature on the impact cancer and associated therapies have on male sexuality, along with identifying gaps in health care providers' knowledge of this topic. Current therapies to treat sexual dysfunction are also presented.

* Corresponding author. School of Nursing, University of Pennsylvania, 418 Curie Boulevard, Philadelphia, PA 19104.
   E-mail address: wbruner@nursing.upenn.edu (D.W. Bruner).

0029-6465/07/$ - see front matter © 2007 Elsevier Inc. All rights reserved.
doi:10.1016/j.cnur.2007.07.005

"Normal" sexual function in males

Physiology of erection

The erectile response is a complex system involving psychologic, bio-chemical, neurologic, and physiologic components. Erection is driven in part by the balance between the nitric oxide stimulus originating from the nonadrenergic, noncholinergic nervous system, and the counterbalancing effect of the sympathetic noradrenergic nerves [1]. The hemodynamics of erection require a delicate balance between pelvic vasculature and muscula-ture and central and peripheral nerves. Mediators of the corpus cavernosum smooth muscle, including adrenergic, cholinergic, and nonadrenergic, non-cholinergic mechanisms are controlled by the central and peripheral nervous systems [1,2].

Sexual response cycle in males

Three major phases of the sexual response cycle have been proposed and include desire, arousal, and orgasm. Desire is the most complex component of the sexual response cycle and consists of the thoughts, fantasies, and feel-ings that are the prelude to engaging in satisfying sexual behaviors. Desire is affected by factors such as fear, anxiety, anger, pain, and body image, as well as disease processes and medications [3]. Desire can be enhanced through touch, visual imagery, and fantasy [4]. Arousal is mediated by the parasympathetic nervous system and is the result of either psychic or so-matic sexual stimulation [5–7]. In males, these nerve impulses cause dilation of the arteries in the penis, causing vasocongestion and consequently erec-tion [5].

Orgasm is mediated by the sympathetic nervous system and is the phys-ical release and peak of pleasurable expression, followed by relaxation [5]. The sympathetic nerves between T12 and L2 control ejaculation [8].

Sexual dysfunction in males

The complexities of the interactions of the systems involved in sexual function described above impress upon us how just one of numerous factors in the pathway of sexual response could mediate ED. In addition, there are distinct gender differences in sexual dysfunction. Males tend to suffer perfor-mance-related disorders (eg, erectile disorder, premature ejaculation), whereas females tend to experience dysfunctions involving desire or satisfac-tion (eg, inhibited sexual desire, inhibited orgasm), with performance disor-ders being relatively infrequent [9].

Male sexual function and aging

Physiologic changes that occur as part of the aging process affect sexual function, particularly erectile function, in men. High levels of ED have been documented in the general population. A large population based study of close to 1,300 subjects between 40 and 70 years of age was conducted to assess "normal" male aging. Increasing age was found to be the most significant independent predictor of ED, although other factors were found to correlate with ED to lesser degrees (e.g., heart disease, hypertension, diabetes, cigarette smoking, among others). Of the subjects in this analysis, 17.2% reported minimal ED, 25.2% reported moderate ED, and 9.6% reported complete ED. The probability of complete ED tripled from 5.1% to 15% in men between 40 and 70 years of age, and the probability of moderate ED doubled from 17% to 34%. An estimated 40% of men age 40 years had minimal, moderate, or complete ED, while that estimate rose to 67% by age 70 years [10].

As cancer is mostly a disease of older age, differentiating age-related versus cancer therapy-related changes in sexual function is can be challenging. It is no surprise that age has been documented as a highly significant predictor of ED post both radical prostatectomy and radiation therapy for prostate cancer [11,12].

Relationships and male sexuality

Several studies have documented the relationship between cancer-related stress and intimacy [13,14], and it is well documented that marital quality and intimacy are related [15,16]. It has also been documented that patients' perceptions of their sexual performance does not match with that of their partners' perception. One study reported the discordance between patient- and partner-rated male sexual performance. Partners reported the patient's ability to have an erection as lower than the patient rated himself, and partners rated the patient's ability to perform sexually worse than the patient rated himself [17].

In a unique study assessing the impact of the difference in patient–partner age and its influence on sexual function post bilateral nerve-sparing radical prostatectomy, it was found that patient age and the age difference between patient and partner were associated with the potency rate following surgery. The mean age and the mean difference in age between patient and partner were approximately 61 and 7 years in the preserved potency group, versus 63 and 4 years in the group with ED, respectively. A greater patient–partner age difference, with partners being on average 7 years younger than the patients, was a significant predictive factor of maintaining postoperative potency independent of patient age [18].

Cancer-related symptoms and sexuality

There are multiple factors associated with the diagnosis and treatment of cancer that have an impact on sexuality, including the complex psychologic and symptom burden of the disease and treatments. While stress and symptoms, such as fatigue and pain, have been documented to interfere with sexual function [14], little research has been devoted to understanding the threshold a particular symptom or combination of symptoms would have to reach to have an impact on intimacy and sexual function. However, it is important for clinicians not to assume that because patients are experiencing symptoms, that all desire for sexual activity is absent in cancer patients. In a rare study assessing sexual functioning and its relationship with psychologic measures in patients with chronic pain, a patient-reported survey was conducted with 70 patients (mean age 50 years) with a mean pain duration of 147 months. Participants experienced a wide variety of pain conditions, yet 66% of patients remained interested in sex. However, only 20% considered their current sexual activity to be adequate, and most were dissatisfied with their orgasms. While over 70% reported that they fantasized at least once a month, only 44% experienced normal arousal during intercourse, 33% practiced masturbation, and 47% were involved in sexual intercourse or oral sex at least once a month. Pain severity, duration, or frequency was not found to be associated with sexual functioning; however, a relationship was found between disability status, age, and several psychologic variables and sexual functioning [19].

Specific cancers and their impact on male sexuality

Prostate cancer

Prostate cancer, the most commonly diagnosed cancer in men, and its associated treatment-related sexual dysfunction has been the subject of a great deal of research over the past decade. As prostate cancer is most common in men aged 65 years or older, distinguishing diagnosis and treatment-related dysfunction from age-related dysfunction becomes even more important in determining cause and effect and potential treatment.

There are several options for the treatment of early stage prostate cancer, with similar efficacy including surgery or radiation therapy. Within each modality there are an increasing number of options, such as nerve-sparing prostatectomy or intensity-modulated radiotherapy (IMRT), each attempting to spare normal tissue effects with similar or improved tumor control. The rates of ED vary widely depending on how the endpoint is measured.

Risk of ED begins with the diagnostic procedures. For example, transurethral resection of the prostate commonly causes retrograde ejaculation and may be associated with a 20% to 50% risk of erectile dysfunction [20–22].

Prostatectomy, even nerve sparing, can cut through the nerves and vasculature required for erectile function. Surgical rates of ED vary by procedure. Stanford and colleagues [23] reported ED rates of 66% in the nonnerve-sparing surgery group, 59% in unilateral surgery group, and 56% in the bilateral nerve-sparing surgery group. Approximately 42% of the men described their sexual performance as a moderate-to-large problem 18 or more months after surgery. Further supporting the importance of assessing sexual outcomes by age, significant differences in sexual function were noted with 39% of men aged less than 60 years, versus 15% to 22% of older men potent at more than 18 months. Furthermore, this study examined racial and ethnic differences in sexual side effects post radical prostatectomy, and found that 38% of black men, 26% of Hispanic men, and 21% of white men reported firm erections at more than 18 months [23].

Although reported rates of ED vary widely among studies, it is clear that patient reported outcomes on self-assessment questionnaires consistently demonstrate higher rates of ED when compared with physician reported ED. For example, several studies assessing patient self-report of sexual function after nerve-sparing radical prostatectomy reported nearly an 80% rate of ED [24,25], far greater than original physician-reported rates of 25% to 58% [26,27].

In addition to ED, radical prostatectomy has been associated with a 50% weakening of the orgasmic sensation. Of concern was a report that 64% of patients had involuntary loss of urine at orgasm, causing more than half to avoid sexual contact with their partner [28]. Penson and colleagues [29] compared sexual outcomes between men with prostate cancer therapy related ED and men with ED related to other etiologies. There was significantly worse sexual self-efficacy, degree of ED, sexual satisfaction, and orgasmic ability for the men treated for prostate cancer. However, men with cancer were psychologically less affected by ED on measures of sexual experience and emotional life.

Radiation therapy can also decrease a man's ability to have voluntary erections, even though desire and sexual sensations may still be present. Although the specific mechanism by which radiation therapy reduces erections is still unknown, it has been suggested that such therapy accelerates atherosclerotic disease, thus interfering with the arterial blood supply of the penis [30]. Current techniques, such as conformal external-beam radiation therapy, may be associated with a 40% to 60% risk of ED [23,31–33]. There had been expectations that newer radiotherapy techniques would be associated with lower rates of ED. However, in recent data from Memorial Sloan Kettering, the 8-year likelihood of ED was 49% among patients with clinically localized prostate cancer treated with IMRT who were potent before treatment [34]. Similar rates of ED were found at the 3-year follow-up after brachytherapy [35].

Hormonal therapy, specifically androgen deprivation, once standard therapy for patients with metastatic prostate cancer, is frequently being used in earlier stage disease. Therapy may consist of monotherapy or combination antiandrogens, such as bicalutamide, nilutamide, or flutamide, and leutenizing hormone-releasing hormone analogs (such as leuprolide to achieve total androgen blockade), estrogen, or bilateral orchiectomy. Antiandrogenic therapies reduce plasma testosterone levels. Very low levels of testosterone are associated with lowered sexual desire, difficulty in achieving a functional erection, less pleasurable orgasm or difficulty in reaching orgasm, decreased semen production, and diminished spermatogenesis [36]. ED rates vary with type of hormonal therapy. For example, ED after orchiectomy alone has been estimated at 47%, for estrogen alone 22%. Total androgen blockade may carry up to an 80% risk of ED [22,37].

The use of hormonal therapy in earlier stage disease and in younger men is especially concerning because of the associated rates of sexual dysfunction. A study by Bruner and colleagues [38] assessed sexual function in younger men (aged 50–65) treated with after radiation therapy, some of whom also had androgen deprivation, as compared with age matched controls. Pretreatment erectile function (sufficient for sexual intercourse) rate for patients was 91%, compared with 85% in age-matched controls. Posttreatment erectile function rates for the radiation therapy-only group was 67%, compared with 41% for the radiotherapy or androgen deprivation therapy group. The radiation therapy-only group was significantly inferior to the control group regarding sexual arousal, function, and frequency, but not in desire or enjoyment. The radiotherapy or androgen deprivation therapy group was significantly inferior to both the control group and the radiation therapy-only group in all areas of sexual functioning measured. The radiotherapy or androgen deprivation therapy group was significantly inferior to the radiotherapy-only group in all areas of sexual functioning measured, even after androgen deprivation therapy was discontinued [38].

Testicular cancer

In the United States, testicular cancer occurs in approximates 6 in every 100,000 men, and mortality rates are 0.4 per 100,000. It is a disease primarily of younger men and occurs most commonly between the ages 20 and 44 years but can occur at even younger ages [39,40]. Sexual dysfunction and infertility are long-lasting sequelae of testicular cancer therapies, affecting approximately 20% of patients [41].

Testicular cancer occurs in young males, whose body image is often devastated by the removal of usually one or sometimes both of their testes. Radical inguinal orchiectomy and lymphadenectomy, which includes removal of the testis, epididymis, a portion of the vas deferens, and the regional lymphatics, interferes with ejaculation, orgasm, and libido, particularly when bilateral [42]. Surgery is usually followed by either radiation therapy or chemotherapy. A study of 123 men in the Netherlands, who had an orchiectomy followed by radiation therapy for Stage I or II testicular seminoma, reported nearly 20% of men had a reduced amount of interest and pleasure in sex and a lower amount of sexual activities, although ED, sexual interest, and satisfaction with sex were not different from age-matched noncancer patients. After the treatment, 17% of the men complained of ED, which was significantly more than before, and this number was correlated with increasing age. Changes in body image were reported by 52% of patients and 32% said their sexual activities were negatively affected by treatment [43]. However, a study by Caffo and colleagues [44] assessing quality of life and sexual function after an orchiectomy and radiotherapy in 98 men with testicular cancer, found only 6% expressed that their body image was worse after the treatment.

Jonker-Pool and colleagues [45] compared nine studies with patients treated for testicular cancer by radiation therapy from 1975 to 2000. They found that men reported multiple areas of sexual dysfunction, including loss of sexual desire (14%), erectile disorder (25%), orgasmic dysfunction (23%), ejaculation disorder (40%), decrease in sexual activity (29%), and sexual dissatisfaction (16%). In contrast, a study of long-time survivors of testicular cancer treated with unilateral orchiectomy and either surveillance or chemotherapy found therapy not to be a risk factor for ED [46].

Penile cancer

Although cancer of the penis is rare, treatment can be devastating and may require partial or total penectomy. Little research has been done in these patients; however, one study assessed sexual function in 14 subjects who had undergone partial penectomy for cancer. Their median age was 50.5 years and the median time of follow-up was 11.5 months. In nine subjects, the overall sexual function was normal or slightly decreased and three subjects had absent sexual function, while 12 subjects reported a slight decrease in sexual satisfaction. Yet, the investigators reported that masculine self-image and the relationship with their partners remained practically unchanged in all of the patients [47].

Colorectal cancer

Rectal cancer surgery has been associated with a high rate of sexual dysfunction because of intraoperative injury or the cutting of the sympathetic or parasympathetic nerves. As with prostate cancer surgery, this has led to experimentation with a nerve-sparing technique, but, as with nerve-sparing radical prostatectomy, a study of this nerve-sparing rectal procedure still reported a high level of ED. Partial to complete ED was observed in 44% of the patients [48]. In a study of sexual function in patients who were part of the United Kingdom Medical Research Council Conventional versus Laparoscopic-Assisted Surgery In Colorectal Cancer trial, outcomes were compared among those who had either a laparoscopic rectal, open rectal, or laparoscopic colonic resection. It was found that laparoscopic rectal resection led to poorer male sexual functioning (erectile and ejaculatory dysfunctioning), although there was also a higher rate of total mesorectal excision (TME) in the laparoscopic rectal resection group [49]. Supporting these findings, Quah and colleagues [50] documented that 46% of sexually active men receiving laparoscopic resection reported ED or impaired ejaculation, compared with only 5% of patients that had an open operation.

TME for rectal cancer appears to cause sexual dysfunction in a third or more of men who were potent before surgery. TME has been reported to lead to decreased sexual desire, ability to have intercourse or orgasm, and less sexual activity [51,52]. However, several small studies have reported high rates of sexual preservation post TME with autonomic nerve preservation [53–55], but these finding require replication in larger samples.

The addition of preoperative radiation therapy to TME has only recently been assessed for its impact on sexual function. Ejaculation and erectile difficulties were found to be significantly greater in men treated with short-term preoperative radiation therapy, as compared with men treated with TME alone. Before preoperative radiation therapy 81% of men were sexually active, but after 24 months this decreased to 67% [56]. Adjuvant radiotherapy and resection was found to have an adverse effect on the ability to get an erection (7.4%), maintain an erection (12.6%), attain an orgasm (16.2%), and be sexually active (13.7%), in comparison with patients undergoing proctosigmoidectomy alone. Maximal deterioration in sexual function was noted at 8 months after surgery followed by slow but not complete recovery [57].

Surgery that includes formation of an ostomy leaves many patients with unique stoma-related sexual concerns. The presence of an ostomy can alter a person's body image, which, in turn, may influence the desire for sexual activity [58]. Body image can be a concern to those acutely aware of their stool collecting visibly in a pouch under their clothing. Fear of embarrassing public and intimate moments because of ostomy appearance, sounds, odors, and leakage can become an obsessive concern to some [42]. Schmidt and colleagues [59] found that abdominoperineal resection and anterior resection with pouch led to poor sexual functioning and that men had more problems with sexual satisfaction. In addition, they found that patients aged 69 and younger had more stress when their sexual function declined, compared with those older than 69 years.

Bladder cancer

There is little documentation of the sexual disruptions for males caused by the diagnosis and treatment of bladder cancer. Early-stage therapy, which usually consists of transurethral resection with or without intravesical chemotherapy, is thought to have a mild, transient effect on sexual functioning. Suprapubic and urethral pain and dyspareunia are possible. Radical cystectomy or external-beam radiation therapy is used in the treatment of invasive bladder cancer [60].

Studies of men post radical cystectomy, and with either an ileal conduit diversion or a modified S-pouch neobladder reconstruction, have reported serious and similar sexual dysfunction. In one study, erections firm enough for intercourse were present in only approximately 18% and 22% of the patients with the ileal conduit or neobladder, respectively [61]. In a study of 40 men who underwent radical cystectomy with ileal conduit urinary diversion, 90% of those who reported they were sexually active before surgery lost the ability to achieve erection following surgery. Although they were unable to achieve penile erection, 41% were able to experience orgasm by means of masturbation [62]. More promising results were found after modified cystectomy in a small series of 10 males who reported sexual function to be fairly well preserved [63].

In a study of sexual function after radiotherapy for bladder cancer, 13 of 18 patients with a 10- to 56-month follow-up, reported being able to achieve an erection before radiotherapy. More than 50% reported a decline in the quality of erections after radiotherapy, with a similar proportion noting decreased libido and frequency of sexual activity. Three patients reported complete ED. Three patients noted reduced frequency of morning erections, five had decreased frequency of ejaculation, and four had reduced intensity of orgasms. The investigators reported that 71% of the patients felt their sex life was worse following radiotherapy but only 56% were concerned about the deterioration [64]. In a study of 37 men (mean age 72 years) treated with bladder conservation therapy (using transurethral resection of the bladder tumor, chemotherapy, and radiation), 39% of men reported no erections in the last 4 weeks, 36% reported full erections, and 18% less firm erections, but sufficient for vaginal penetration. A total of 54% were capable of orgasm and 50% of ejaculation. Only 8% of men reported they were dissatisfied with their sex life, while 59% were satisfied, and 33% were neither satisfied nor dissatisfied. Five of the men reported using sildenafil to assist with erections [65].

Head and neck cancer

Cancers that do not directly affect sexual organs may have no less an impact on sexual self-image, and indeed the cluster of symptoms associated with cancers often have a cumulative detrimental effect on sexual function. Head and neck cancers may be treated with disfiguring surgery, affecting body image. Radiation therapy used in the treatment of head and neck cancers may cause permanent xerostomia, affecting comfort and libido and impairing the ability for oral sexual contact. To put this in context, oral-genital contact (cunnilingus) rose from 51%, in the classic Kinsey sample of the 1940s, to 69% of nonvirgin adolescents (both males and females) and 87% of adults by the 1980s [66,67]. This underscores the importance of this activity as a normal sexual behavior and raises concerns for the lack of clinician attention to disease and treatment related symptoms that interfere with the oral mucosa.

Decrease in the ability to function sexually does not correlate with continued interest in sexual activity. In a study of 55 head and neck cancer patients following radiation therapy with or without surgery, 85% reported continued interested in sex, although the majority reported arousal problems and 58% had orgasmic problems. Almost 60% no longer had intercourse, yet 49% reported being satisfied with their current sexual functioning [19,68].

It is not only the ravages of surgery and radiotherapy that impact sexual function in patients treated with head and neck cancer. Roberge and colleagues [69] found that one third of patients who had home enteral tube feeding because of head and neck or esophageal cancer did not like their body image. In addition, 15% did not visit family or have close relationships and 23% would not be seen in public because of the tube. It is not difficult to imagine the high rates of sexual dysfunction associated with these concerns for body image, and deterioration of relationships.

Other influences

Fatigue and loss of energy appear to negatively impact sexual function in a number of cancers, including lung cancer and Hodgkin's disease [70,71]. Sexual dysfunction has also been documented with the treatment of sarcomas. Whether limb-amputation or limb-sparing radical radiation therapy is used, high rates of posttreatment sexual dysfunction have been noted. In one study, 47% of subjects reported decreased sexual frequency, although another 13% reported increased frequency at 6-months post treatment compared with pretreatment. At 12 months posttherapy, almost half of the subjects reported decreased frequency and decreased interest in sexual activity [72]. It had been assumed that limb-sparing therapy would improve sexual function, compared with amputation, but studies have not been able to substantiate this hypothesis [72,73].

Assessment of sexual function

Sexuality should be routinely assessed, as other body systems, by the nurse or physician in the process of taking a health history. Routinizing sexual assessment helps decrease any initial discomfort for the practitioner and indicates to the patient that sexuality is a normal human function and just as valid for discussion as any other bodily function.

The sexual history

General aspects of the sexual history are discussed in other articles in this edition. Table 1 [10,74–81] presents specific issues related to taking the male sexual history.

Specific sexual questions to ask

Clinicians often request specific suggestions regarding questions to ask about sexuality. The following are a number of suggestions, beginning

Table 1
Taking a sexual history in the male cancer patient

History	Evaluation
Cancer diagnosis	Prognostic factors, like extent of disease invasion into sexual tissue, and the therapeutic plan and expected side effects, such as the impact of surgery on erectile vasculature, will have bearing on ED.
Age	There are normal physiologic changes that occur with age which increase risk of ED by decade, as described above and in further detail elsewhere [74–76].
Sexual orientation	ED should be assessed in context, and health care professionals must be prepared to assess and respect the individual's sexual orientation [77,78].
Cultural and ethnic background	The meaning and degree of significance ED has related to male sexuality varies among cultures and religions; and it is important for the clinician to be aware of the issues related to their particular patient population [10,79].
Concomitant chronic illness	Diseases that effect the muscular, neurologic, or vascular systems (eg, diabetes, hypertension, arthritis, urologic problems) compound the risk of ED with cancer therapy.
Medications	Many classes of pharmaceuticals and recreational drugs, including antihypertensives, antipsychotics, antidepressants, opiates, cocaine, tobacco, marijuana, sedatives, and alcohol decrease libido and increase ED [80].
Preillness sexual functioning	This has been found to be a significant predictor of posttreatment functioning. In general, men who had good sexual performance pretreatment are more likely to have acceptable sexual outcomes posttreatment [81].

with general questions and moving on to more specific questions. The need to delve into more specific detail depends on the level of sexual function the patient is experiencing and the level of clinician comfort. Communication will be facilitated if the practitioner uses bridge statements to transition from comfortable topics to those that are less comfortable. An example of a bridge question and a good way to initiate the discussion is, "Has the quality of intercourse or sexual contact changed since your cancer treatment?"

Specific sexual questions to include in a health history

- Has the quality of intercourse or sexual contact changed since your cancer treatment?
    - If yes, in what way?
    - Do you have any problems with having erections?
    - If yes continue... Do you have erections firm enough for intercourse?

- Do you awaken in the morning with an erection?
- Do you have problems with ejaculation?
- Have you tried an erectile aide?
  ○ If so, what type and how well has it worked for you?
- Are you satisfied with your level of sexual function?

Diagnostic evaluation

Although there are a variety of physiologic measures available to assess erectile dysfunction [82,83], they predominantly focus on differentiation of psychogenic versus organic etiologies, and are usually not indicated in treating ED post cancer therapy. Patient self-report of pre- or posttreatment changes in erectile and overall sexual function is the most appropriate evaluation in cancer patients to date. Testosterone levels can be measured; however, they have poor correlation with sexual function and the dose-response relationship between plasma testosterone levels and ED remains unclear [46].

Treatments of sexual dysfunction

Pharmacologic and nonpharmacologic interventions are available that can restore voluntary erectile function for sexual intercourse. The approval of the class of phosphodiesterase type 5 (PDE5) inhibitor medications, in particular, have revolutionized the treatment of ED. These oral agents work by releasing nitrous oxide, which inhibits PDE5, causing increased levels of cyclic guanosine monophosphate, which in turn enhances smooth muscle relaxation and inflow of blood in the corpus cavernosum. This occurs in conjunction with sexual stimulation. Efficacy data has shown that there are similar improvements in erectile function among the current FDA approved PDE5 inhibitors, sildenafil, vardenafil, and tadalafil. More important than which therapy is used to improve ED, is the emerging evidence that early institution of treatment for ED may promote improvement in the return of spontaneous erections after cancer therapy [84–87].

Regardless of the type, reports indicate a high number of men seek remedies for ED. Stephenson and colleagues [88] found that nearly half of the men in their study used ED treatment within 5 years after their prostate cancer diagnosis and treatment with either radical prostatectomy or external beam radiation therapy. However, there was only a modest improvement in men who used treatment when compared with men who did not have treatment at the 5-year time frame. This low rate of success of many of these ED treatments was confirmed in a larger study of over 1,200 men after radical prostatectomy where, even with erectile aides, only 28% reported erections sufficient for intercourse at 5-years post surgery. The most common ED therapies reported were sildenafil (used by 43% of men), penile prosthesis (4%), vacuum constriction device (25%), intracavernous injection (17%), some other aid (alprostadil, yohimbine, and others, 7%), and psychotherapy (4%) [24].

Pharmacotherapies

Sildenafil

Sildenafil citrate (Viagra) has been taken by more than 20 million men in more than 110 countries. Across a variety of etiologies there are reports as high as an 82% success rate in users. However, specifically related to cancer, there is about a 43% success rate in users that had a radical prostatectomy, as compared with 15% to 20% with placebo [89]. In an initial series of patients treated with radiotherapy for prostate cancer on open-label, non-randomized trials using small convenience samples, an improved response in erections was seen in approximately 70% to 80% of patients, about twice the rate Pfizer reported after radical prostatectomy [90–93]. However, in the first double-blinded randomized trial of sildenafil in subjects treated with radiotherapy, the positive response rate was 55%, closer to the randomized radical prostatectomy reports than the nonrandomized earlier radiotherapy studies [94]. Whether the erectile dysfunction is caused by prostate cancer, diabetes, or psychogenic reasons, the drug is thought to be effective and safe for those even with coronary artery disease (as long as nitrates aren't used). Headaches, flushing, and dyspepsia are the most common negative side effects [95]. The pill is usually taken within 1 hour before intercourse; however, the onset of action for sildenafil can be as short as 20 minutes and the duration of action may be as long as 18 hours [96]. Dosage and duration of action of each of the PDE5 inhibitors is displayed in Table 2.

Vardenafil

As with sildenafil, vardenafil (Levitra) has shown significant effects, when compared with a placebo, in patients with cancer related ED [97,98]. In a study by Nehra and colleagues [98], men treated with nerve-sparing radical retropubic prostatectomy showed improved intercourse satisfaction, orgasmic function, hardness of erection, and overall satisfaction during the sexual encounter in those treated with vardenafil. Side effects include headache, vasodilation, and rhinitis. Vardenafil appears to have similar effectiveness in patients treated with cancer as compared with sildenafil; however, vardenafil does not affect color perception, which may occur in a small percentage of patients treated with sildenafil.

Tadalafil

Tadalafil, (Cialis) has an extended period of effectiveness, up to 36 hours, and while it appears to have similar efficacy to sildenafil and vardenafil, men appear to prefer the longer duration of effect. One study of men who were using sildenafil, then switched to tadalafil, found that men preferred to remain on tadalafil by a ratio of nine to one. However, there were limitations

Table 2
Dosage, duration of effect and special instructions for 3 PDE5-inhibitors for the treatment of ED

Generic name	Trade name	Dosages available	Usual dose reported as effective in cancer patients	Time to take effect	Duration of effect	Special instructions
Sildenafil	Viagra	25 mg, 50 mg, 100 mg	100 mg [94]	30 min	4 hours	To get the quickest results, avoid high-fat meals 2 hours before[a]
Vardenafil	Levitra	2.5 mg, 5 mg, 10 mg, 20 mg	20 mg [97]	30 min	4–5 hours[b]	May be taken with or without meals[b]
Tadalafil	Cialis	5 mg, 10 mg, 20 mg	20 mg [102]	30 min	up to 36 hours	May be taken with or without meals[c]

[a] http://www.viagra.com/content/how-to-take-viagra.jsp?setShowOn=../content/taking-viagra. jsp&setShowHighlightOn=../content/how-to-take-viagra.jsp.
[b] http://www.univgraph.com/bayer/inserts/levitra.pdf.
[c] http://www.cialis.com/about_cialis/02_02.jsp?reqNavId=1.4.

to the study that included different dosage levels and different dosage instructions [99]. Preference for tadalafil is most likely because of the longer amount of time of its effectiveness as compared with sildenafil and vardenafil.

As the newest PDE5 inhibitor to be FDA approved, few randomized trials of this drug have yet to be conducted in patients with prostate cancer. There are two randomized studies in the literature assessing tadalafil for the improvement of ED after radical prostatectomy. In one study, 4,262 subjects were randomized to either on-demand or three-times-per-week dosage regimens of tadalafil 20 mg. Either was equally efficacious in returning those with ED to normal erectile function (60% and 62% of subjects reported normal erectile function scores, respectively) [100]. In a second study, a total of 303 men (mean age 60 years) with preoperative normal erectile function, who had undergone a bilateral nerve-sparing radical retropubic prostatectomy 12 to 48 months before the study, were randomized (2:1) to tadalafil, (20 mg on demand; n = 201) or placebo (102). For all subjects who received tadalafil, the mean percentage of successful penetration attempts was 54%, and the mean percentage of successful intercourse attempts was 41%. Of all the patients randomized to tadalafil, 62% reported improved erections. Patients receiving tadalafil reported greater treatment satisfaction than those receiving placebo. The most commonly reported side effects were mild and included headache (21%), dyspepsia (13%), and myalgia (7%) [101].

There is one additional randomized study in the literature assessing tadalafil for the improvement of ED after radiotherapy. Sixty patients who completed three-dimensional conformal external-beam radiotherapy at least 12 months before the study were entered on a double-blind, placebo-controlled, cross-over study lasting 12 weeks. They received 20 mg of on-demand tadalafil or placebo for 6 weeks and then switched to the alternative. Mean age at study entry was 69 years. Outcomes were significantly improved with tadalafil, with 67% of the subjects reporting an improvement of erectile function with tadalafil, versus 20% with placebo, and 48% reporting successful intercourse with tadalafil, versus 9% with placebo [102].

Testosterone replacement

Testosterone replacement is not an option for hormone-sensitive prostate cancer. However, many practitioners question its use in other cancers. The involvement of testosterone in erectile response is not as straightforward as some may think and usually, other than those with congenital deficiencies, testosterone replacement has shown poor efficacy in improving erectile dysfunction. One study examined the effect of intramuscular injections with testosterone on sexual functioning in seven subjects treated with orchiectomy for bilateral testicular cancer. After injection there was a rapid decline of plasma testosterone to levels below the lower normal limit. Sexual functioning was not improved with the injections; rather, at the end of the injection interval, adverse psychologic and physical effects had a significant impact on libido and arousal [103].

Other agents

Just before FDA approval of sildenafil, the American Urologic Association (AUA) Clinical Guidelines Panel on ED, published recommendations based on the treatment outcomes data on men with organic (versus psychologic) ED. The panel reviewed published outcomes for five treatment alternatives, including intracavernous vasoactive agents, vacuum constriction devices, penile prosthesis implants, venous and arterial surgery, and oral drug therapy with yohimbine. The panel concluded that only the first three alternatives had acceptable outcomes in terms of return to intercourse, patient satisfaction, and partner satisfaction [104].

Although PDE5 inhibitors have revolutionized the treatment of erectile dysfunction, there remain patients who fail to respond to these medications. For these men, alternative treatment with intracavernous prostaglandin E1 injection therapy, which is thought to reduce the incidence of veno-occlusive dysfunction, transurethral alprostadil, and combination therapy is available. These therapies have been shown to improve penile rigidity. Intracavernous injection therapy and transurethral alprostadil are highly effective in the management of postprostatectomy ED. However, high dropout rates, unrelated to adverse effects, have been described with both modalities [84,105]. A self-care guide for self-injection of prostaglandin for ED is available, which may enhance at least initial use of this therapy [60].

Transurethral alprostadil, also known as the medicated urethral system for erection (MUSE), has been shown to have approximately a 40% success rate for sexual intercourse following radical prostatectomy when used alone [106]. However, combined with sildenafil, MUSE treatment of erectile dysfunction following nerve-sparing radical prostatectomy demonstrated an 80% improvement with the penile rigidity, intercourse, and sexual satisfaction in a small sample of patients (n = 23). All patients started on 100 mg, 1 hour before intercourse of oral sildenafil more than 6 months after radical prostatectomy. Patients used combination therapy for a minimum of four attempts before assessment [107].

Vacuum constriction devices

Vacuum constriction devices make use of hollow tube, placed around the flaccid penis, which are manually pumped to create a negative pressure. Arterial blood inflow, as well as venous backflow, fills the corpora cavernosa [108]. When a rigid erection is achieved, an elastic constriction band is placed around the base of the penis to preserve the rigidity and allow for vaginal or anal penetration. The constriction may be maintained for up to 30 minutes. Although the device may be used daily, penile bruising and ischemia can occur with excessive use.

Vacuum constriction devices have shown efficacy following radical prostatectomy. In 109 patients who were treated with either nerve-sparing or nonnerve-sparing surgery for prostate cancer, those randomized to the device for 9 months of daily use showed an 80% (60/74) success rate for vaginal intercourse at a frequency of twice a week, as compared with those randomized to the no ED therapy arm. After 9 months of use, 32% (19/60) of patients reported return of natural erections, but only 17% had natural erections sufficient for vaginal penetration [87].

Surgical therapies

Three types of penile prostheses are available: semirigid, semi-inflatable, and fully inflatable prostheses. The semirigid prosthesis is easy to surgically insert and to use. Two solid silicone rods are placed into the corpora cavernosa. These rods are firm yet bendable, and allow for vaginal or anal penetration. However, they leave the patient with a permanent erection. The erection may be concealed by positioning the penis up against the abdomen and securing it with briefs; however, rod breakage is possible and would render the prosthesis useless.

The semi- and fully-inflatable prostheses require more intensive surgical insertions, and basically consist of two cylinders which are placed into the corpora cavernosa. These are attached to a pump and reservoir system. The patient or partner must manually pump the fluid (usually saline) from the reservoir to the cylinders. The pump is usually behind the glans penis, for the semi-inflatable, or in the scrotal sac for the fully inflatable device. To deflate the semi-inflatable device, the patient holds down the penis for about 10 seconds to allow the fluid to return to the reservoir. The advantage of the semi-inflatable prosthesis is that full erections are possible with no permanent erection. However, although the penis is more concealable, it never becomes totally flaccid. For the fully inflatable device, the pump is squeezed to move the fluid from the reservoir to the cylinders in the penis, and to return the fluid to the reservoir the release valve is pressed in the scrotal sac. Both devices allow for firm but not permanent erections, as with the semi-rigid device. However, with the semi-inflatable device, the penis is never totally flaccid and it does not increase girth, whereas the fully inflatable prosthesis produces more natural erections, with an increased penile girth and total flaccidity when not erect [60].

Penile prostheses have been shown to improve sexual function in men treated with radical prostatectomy, radiation therapy, or the combination [85,109].

Complimentary and alternative therapies

Throughout history, men have sought remedies to enhance normal sexual function and treat sexual dysfunction. Much of what we now call "alternative" or "complementary" medicines have been used by numerous cultures over the centuries. However, despite long years of use and anecdotal reports of improvements in sexual function, scientific evidence is slim if not entirely lacking for many of these treatments. These complementary therapies include plants and herbs and non-Western approaches, such as traditional Chinese medicine and acupuncture.

Plants and herbs

The list of plants and herbs and other items that have been purported to improve ED around the globe is too lengthy to mention, but a few examples include such things as elephant tusks, lion blood, bull testicles, rhino horn, deer antlers, ram penis, and pig genitals [110]. Further, advertisements for herbal treatments for erectile dysfunction abound. However, extreme caution must be used. If any work, they may work by increasing levels of unbound (free) testosterone, which could stimulate prostate cancer cell growth.

On the other hand, patients with cancers other than prostate, and a normal prostate specific antigen level and prostate exam, may be able to take herbal supplements as long at the patient's physician is aware of the use.

One plant extract that has actually been the focus of considerable research is yohimbe. The mechanism by which this compound improves ED is not fully understood. It has been proposed that inhibition of central α-adrenoceptors, which decrease neuro-sympathetic tone and blood pressure by antagonists such as yohimbe, results in an increase in sympathetic tone and an increase in blood pressure to the penis [2]. However, it appears that if this plant extract from the bark of the *Pausinystalia yohimbe* tree, is active for erectile dysfunction, it is minimal, and with the advent of PDE5 inhibitors and other more effective therapies, it is no longer recommended by medical professionals for the treatment of ED [104,111]. Yet despite recommendations from the AUA and other investigators against use of yohimbe for ED, research continues with this compound alone and in combination with other compounds, such as L-arginine glutamate, and small pilot studies continue to report promising results [112,113]. The amino acid arginine produces nitrous oxide, one of the primary mediators of erection during its metabolism. Although randomized studies have generally not found arginine to be active, it may be that men who are nitrous oxide deficient (as measured in the urine) respond to arginine supplementation [114].

Ginseng (*Panax ginseng*) is an herb thought in traditional Chinese medicine to improve potency by increasing the body's ability to handle environmental stresses, decrease fatigue, and control anxiety [2]. However, more evidence-based research shows that ginseng acts by increasing penile vasodilatation and relaxation of the corpus cavernosum by the release of nitric oxide [115]. Several small trials have shown improvements in erectile response with the Korean red ginseng [116]. However, a major concern with the use of ginseng after prostate cancer is that it may also increase sex-related hormones, such as testosterone.

Traditional Chinese medicine

Traditional Chinese medicine, still actively taught and practiced around the world, is a complex system that is primarily based on the balance of the energy components, the yin and the yang, of the body. Yang represents the hot, or active aspects of the body, whereas the yin represents the cold, or passive aspects of the body. Sexual dysfunction is thought to be a yang deficiency, with cold blocking blood flow to the genital region. Methods of treatment can include acupuncture or ingestion of specific foods and herbs, such as ginseng [60].

Acupuncture

Acupuncture for erectile dysfunction has been tested prospectively and, as with other alternative therapies, found to be effective in small non-randomized trials. In one study of 29 subjects, 70% reported increased ability to have an erection after acupuncture [117]. In a second study of 16 subjects, 40% reported improvement in erectile function [118].

Counseling

Some degree of sexual dysfunction may be temporary or permanent after many types of cancers faced by men. Nevertheless, sexual counseling is not routinely provided in most oncology treatment settings. Most patients and their partners can benefit from brief counseling that includes education on the impact of cancer treatment on sexual functioning, recommendations on when to resume sexual activity, and specific suggestions on resuming sex comfortably. Most couples would benefit from learning to improve communication about sexual needs and concerns. Counseling could be advantageous in motivating couples to improve sexual communications and correct common mistakes in the use of erectile medication administration or erectile aides. Many patients would benefit from advice on how to mitigate the effects of physical handicaps, (such as having an ostomy) on sexuality, and self-help strategies to manage specific cancer related side-effects that may interfere with sexual function, such as pain or fatigue. Brief counseling can be provided by the treating physician, the nurse, or one of the allied health professionals on the oncology treatment team. Some patients will need specialized, intensive medical or psychologic treatment for a sexual dysfunction, and it is best for the nurse to be prepared with appropriate referrals, as needed. Overall, counseling would likely improve treatment efficacy, compliance, and decrease dropout rates [78].

In telephone interviews with 320 prostate cancer survivors, who had previously reported on a survey that they were likely to seek help in the next year for a sexual problem, most were found to have had difficulty in finding assistance with their ED. Men in this study preferred to seek help from a urologist or prostate cancer specialist for ED, and most preferred an oral agent to other methods of erectile aides. Although 91% had tried to find medical help, sadly, most reported their attempts remained unsuccessful [119]. Although there is a dearth of research devoted to assessing the impact of professional counseling on sexual functioning after cancer therapy, two recent studies have shown promise. One study assessed the utility of sexual counseling after nonnerve-sparing radical prostatectomy or cystectomy in 57 subjects treated with prostaglandin E1 intracavernous injections. The group receiving the additional sexual counseling had statistically higher scores on measures of sexual satisfaction, sexual desire, orgasmic function, and general satisfaction. At the end of follow-up, 21 subjects in the counseling group, versus 12 in the no-counseling group, reported satisfaction with treatment [120].

A second study examined a four session counseling program that was intended to help increase sexual satisfaction and knowledge of ED treatment for 51 prostate cancer survivors and their partners. At the 3-month follow-up there was a 31% increase in usage of ED treatment, and a 49% increase at the 6-month follow-up. In addition, after 3 months, couples reported improvement with male and female global sexual function and with male distress, but this trend regressed toward the baseline after 6 months [121].

Summary

Cancers and the therapies used to treat them have a well-documented and significant negative impact on sexual function. There are an increasing number of remedies available to treat erectile dysfunction in men; however, success rates are variable and long-term compliance is generally low. Early intervention, combination therapy—as opposed to monotherapy—and the addition of even brief sexual counseling may improve sexual outcomes for men with cancer.

References

[1] Traish AM, Kim NN, Goldstein I, et al. Alpha-adrenergic receptors in the penis: identification, characterization, and physiological function. J Androl 1999;20(6):671–82.

[2] Tam SW, Worcel M, Wyllie M. Yohimbine: a clinical review. Pharmacol Ther 2001;91(3): 215–43.

[3] Wilmoth M, Bruner DW. Including sexuality into cancer nursing practice: tips and techniques. Oncology Nursing Updates 2002;9(1):1–14.

[4] Nutter DE, Condron MK. Sexual fantasy and activity patterns of males with inhibited sexual desire and males with erectile dysfunction versus normal controls. J Sex Marital Ther 1985;11(2):91–8.

[5] Guyton AC. Basic neuroscience: anatomy and physiology. 2nd edition. Philadelphia: Saunders; 1992.

[6] Masters WH, Johnson VE. Human sexual response. Boston: Little, Brown, and Company; 1966.

[7] Sands JK. Human sexuality. In: Phipps WJ, Cassmeyer VL, Sands JK, et al, editors. Medical surgical nursing: concepts and clinical practice. 5th edition. St. Louis (MO): Mosby; 1995. p. 262–84.

[8] Koukouras D, Spiliotis J, Scopa C, et al. Radical consequence in the sexuality of male patients operated for colorectal carcinoma. Eur J Surg Oncol 1991;17:285–8.

[9] Derogatis L. Article review: how cancer affects sexual functioning. Oncology 1990;4(6): 92–3.

[10] Feldman HA, Goldstein I, Hatzichristou DG, et al. Impotence and its medical and psychosocial correlates: results of the Massachusetts male aging study. J Urol 1994;151:54–61.

[11] Bruner DW, Scott C, McGowan D, et al. Factors influencing sexual outcomes in prostate cancer patients enrolled on Radiation Therapy Oncology Group (RTOG) studies 90-20 and 94-08 [abstract]. Paper presented at the 5th Annual Conference of The International Society for Quality of Life Research (ISOQOL). Baltimore (MD); November 15–17, 1998.

[12] Karakiewicz PI, Tanguay S, Kattan MW, et al. Erectile and urinary dysfunction after radical prostatectomy for prostate cancer in Quebec: a population-based study of 2415 men. Eur Urol 2004;46(2):188–94.

[13] Banthia R, Malcarne VL, Varni JW, et al. The effects of dyadic strength and coping styles on psychological distress in couples faced with prostate cancer. J Behav Med 2003;26(1): 31–52.

[14] Gaugler JE, Hanna N, Linder J, et al. Cancer caregiving and subjective stress: a multi-site, multi-dimensional analysis. Psychooncology 2005;14(9):771–85.

[15] Eton DT, Lepore SJ, Helgeson VS. Psychological distress in spouses of men treated for early-stage prostate carcinoma. Cancer 2005;103(11):2412–8.

[16] Johnson JE, Fieler VK, Wlasowicz GS, et al. The effects of nursing care guides by self-regulation theory on coping with radiation therapy. Oncol Nurs Forum 1997;24(6):1041–50.

[17] Soloway CT, Soloway MS, Kim SS, et al. Sexual, psychological and dyadic qualities of the prostate cancer 'couple'. BJU Int 2005;95(6):780–5.

[18] Descazeaud A, Debre B, Flam TA. Age difference between patient and partner is a predictive factor of potency rate following radical prostatectomy. J Urol 2006;176(6 Pt 1):2594–8.

[19] Monga TN, Tan G, Ostermann HJ, et al. Sexuality and sexual adjustment of patients with chronic pain. Disabil Rehabil 1998;20(9):317–29.

[20] Bieri S, Miralbell R, Rohner S, et al. Influence of transurethral resection on sexual dysfunction in patients with prostate cancer. Br J Urol 1996;78(4):537–41.

[21] Deliveliotis C, Liakouras C, Delis A, et al. Prostate operations: long-term effects on sexual and urinary function and quality of life. Comparison with an age-matched control population. Urol Res 2004;32(4):283–9.

[22] Schover LR. Sexual rehabilitation after treatment for prostate cancer. Cancer 1993; 72(3 Suppl):1024–30.

[23] Stanford JL, Feng Z, Hamilton AS, et al. Urinary and sexual function after radical prostatectomy for clinically localized prostate cancer: the Prostate Cancer Outcomes Study. J Am Med Assoc 2000;283(3):354–60.

[24] Penson DF, McLerran D, Feng Z, et al. 5-year urinary and sexual outcomes after radical prostatectomy: results from the prostate cancer outcomes study. J Urol 2005;173(5): 1701–5.

[25] Talcott JA, Rieker P, Propert KJ, et al. Patient-reported impotence and incontinence after nerve-sparing radical prostatectomy. J Natl Cancer Inst 1997;89(15):1117–23.

[26] Banker FL. The preservation of potency after external beam irradiation for prostate cancer. Int J Radiat Oncol Biol Phys 1988;15(1):219–20.

[27] Walsh PC. Radical prostatectomy, preservation of sexual function, cancer control: the controversy. Urol Clin North Am 1987;14(4):663–73.

[28] Koeman M, vD MF, Schultz WC, et al. Orgasm after radical prostatectomy. Br J Urol 1996;77(6):861–4.

[29] Penson DF, Latini DM, Lubeck DP, et al. Is quality of life different for men with erectile dysfunction and prostate cancer compared to men with erectile dysfunction due to other causes? Results from the ExCEED data base. J Urol 2003;169(4):1458–61.

[30] Goldstein I, Feldman M, Deckers P, et al. Radiation associated impotence: a clinical study of its mechanism. J Am Med Assoc 1984;251:903–10.

[31] Jonler M, Ritter MA, Brinkmann R, et al. Sequelae of definitive radiation therapy for prostate cancer localized to the pelvis. Urology 1994;44(6):876–82.

[32] Kao TC, Cruess DF, Garner D, et al. Multicenter patient self-reporting questionnaire on impotence, incontinence and stricture after radical prostatectomy. J Urol 2000;163(3): 858–64.

[33] Talcott J, Rieker P, Propert K, et al. Long-term complications of treatment for early prostate cancer: 2-year follow-up in a prospective, multi-institutional outcomes study [abstract]. Proc Am Soc Clinical Oncol 1996;15:252.

[34] Zelefsky MJ, Chan H, Hunt M, et al. Long-term outcome of high dose intensity modulated radiation therapy for patients with clinically localized prostate cancer. J Urol 2006; 176(4 Pt 1):1415–9.

[35] Merrick GS, Butler WM, Wallner KE, et al. Erectile function after prostate brachytherapy. Int J Radiat Oncol Biol Phys 2005;62(2):437–47.

[36] Smith D, Babaian R. The effects of treatment for cancer on male fertility and sexuality. Cancer Nurs 1992;15(4):271–5.

[37] Rousseau L, Dupont A, Labrie F, et al. Sexuality changes in prostate cancer patients receiving antihormonal therapy combining the anti-androgen flutamide with medical (LHRH Agonist) or surgical castration. Arch Sex Behav 1988;17(1):87–98.

[38] Bruner DW, Hanlon A, Nicolaou N, et al. Sexual function after radiotherapy ± androgen deprivation for clinically localized prostate cancer in younger men (age 50–65) [abstract]. Oncol Nurs Forum 1997;24(2):327.

[39] Bertuccio P, Malvezzi M, Chatenoud L, et al. Testicular cancer mortality in the Americas, 1980–2003. Cancer 2007;109(4):776–9.

[40] McGlynn KA, Devesa SS, Graubard BI, et al. Increasing incidence of testicular germ cell tumors among black men in the United States. J Clin Oncol 2005;23(24):5757–61.

[41] Kuczyk M, Machtens S, Bokemeyer C, et al. Sexual function and fertility after treatment of testicular cancer. Curr Opin Urol 2000;10(5):473–7.

[42] Bruner DW, Iwamato R. Altered sexuality. In: Groenwald S, Frogge M, Goodman M, et al, editors. Cancer symptom management. 2nd edition. Boston: Jones and Bartlett; 1999.

[43] Incrocci L, Hop WC, Wijnmaalen A, et al. Treatment outcome, body image, and sexual functioning after orchiectomy and radiotherapy for Stage I-II testicular seminoma. Int J Radiat Oncol Biol Phys 2002;53(5):1165–73.

[44] Caffo O, Amichetti M, Tomio L, et al. Quality of life after radiotherapy for early-stage testicular seminoma. Radiother Oncol 2001;59(1):13–20.

[45] Jonker-Pool G, Van de Wiel HB, Hoekstra HJ, et al. Sexual functioning after treatment for testicular cancer—review and meta-analysis of 36 empirical studies between 1975–2000. Arch Sex Behav 2001;30(1):55–74.

[46] Lackners J, Schatzl G, Koller A, et al. Treatment of testicular cancer: influence on pituitary-gonadal axis and sexual function. Urology 2005;66(2):402–6.

[47] D'Ancona CA, Botega NJ, DeMoraes C, et al. Quality of life after partial penectomy for penile carcinoma. Urology 1997;50(4):593–6.

[48] Mancini R, Cosimelli M, Filippini A, et al. Nerve-sparing surgery in rectal cancer: feasibility and functional results. J Exp Clin Cancer Res 2000;19(1):35–40.

[49] Jayne DG, Brown JM, Thorpe H, et al. Bladder and sexual function following resection for rectal cancer in a randomized clinical trial of laparoscopic versus open technique. Br J Surg 2005;92(9):1124–32.

[50] Quah HM, Jayne DG, Eu KW, et al. Bladder and sexual dysfunction following laparoscopically assisted and conventional open mesorectal resection for cancer. Br J Surg 2002; 89(12):1551–6.

[51] Maurer CA, Z'Graggen K, Renzulli P, et al. Total mesorectal excision preserves male genital function compared with conventional rectal cancer surgery. Br J Surg 2001;88(11): 1501–5.

[52] Sterk P, Shekarriz B, Gunter S, et al. Voiding and sexual dysfunction after deep rectal resection and total mesorectal excision: prospective study on 52 patients. Int J Colorectal Dis 2005;20(5):423–7.

[53] Kim NK, Aahn TW, Park JK, et al. Assessment of sexual and voiding function after total mesorectal excision with pelvic autonomic nerve preservation in males with rectal cancer. Dis Colon Rectum 2002;45(9):1178–85.

[54] Nesbakken A, Nygaard K, Bull-Njaa T, et al. Bladder and sexual dysfunction after mesorectal excision for rectal cancer. Br J Surg 2000;87(2):206–10.

[55] Pocard M, Zinzindohoue F, Haab F, et al. A prospective study of sexual and urinary function before and after total mesorectal excision with autonomic nerve preservation for rectal cancer. Surgery 2002;131(4):368–72.

[56] Marijnen CA, van de Velde CJ, Putter H, et al. Impact of short-term preoperative radiotherapy on health-related quality of life and sexual functioning in primary rectal cancer: report of a multicenter randomized trial. J Clin Oncol 2005;23(9): 1847–58.

[57] Heriot AG, Tekkis PP, Fazio VW, et al. Adjuvant radiotherapy is associated with increased sexual dysfunction in male patients undergoing resection for rectal cancer: a predictive model. Ann Surg 2005;242(4):502–10.

[58] Sprunk E, Alteneder RR. The impact of an ostomy on sexuality. Clin J Oncol Nurs 2000; 42(2):85–8.

[59] Schmidt CE, Bestmann B, Kuchler T, et al. Factors influencing sexual function in patients with rectal cancer. Int J Impot Res 2005;17(3):231–8.

[60] Bruner DW, Berk L. Altered body image and sexual health. In: Yarbro C, Frogge M, Goodman M, editors. In Cancer symptom management. 3rd edition. Boston: Jones and Bartlett; 2003. p. 596–603.

[61] Protogerou V, Moschou M, Antoniou N, et al. Modified S-pouch neobladder vs ileal conduit and a matched control population: a quality-of-life survey. BJU Int 2004;94(3):350–4.

[62] Nordstrom GM, Nyman CR. Male and female sexual function and activity following ileal conduit urinary diversion. Br J Urol 1992;70(1):33–9.

[63] Horenblas S, Meinhardt W, Ijzerman W, et al. Sexuality preserving cystectomy and neobladder: initial results. J Urol 2001;166(3):837–40.

[64] Little FA, Howard GC. Sexual function following radical radiotherapy for bladder cancer. Radiother Oncol 1998;49(2):157–61.

[65] Zietman AL, Sacco D, Skowronski U, et al. Organ conservation in invasive bladder cancer by transurethral resection, chemotherapy and radiation: results of a urodynamic and quality of life study on long-term survivors. J Urol 2003;170(5):1781–2.

[66] Newcomer SF, Udry JR. Oral sex in an adolescent population. Arch Sex Behav 1985;14(1): 41–6.

[67] Wyatt GE, Peters SD, Guthrie D. Kinsey revisited, Part I: comparisons of the sexual socialization and sexual behavior of white women over 33 years. Arch Sex Behav 1988;17(3): 201–39.

[68] Monga U, Tan G, Ostermann H, et al. Sexuality in the head and neck cancer patient. Arch Phys Med Rehabil 1997;78:298–304.

[69] Roberge C, Tran M, Massoud C, et al. Quality of life and home enteral tube feeding: a French prospective study in patients with head and neck or oesophageal cancer. Br J Cancer 2000;82(2):263–9.

[70] Kornblith AB, Herndon JE 2nd, Zuckerman E, et al. Comparison of psychosocial adaptation of advanced stage Hodgkin's disease and acute leukemia survivors. Ann Oncol 1998; 9(3):297–306.

[71] Schimmer AD, Stewart AK, Imrie K, et al. Male sexual function after autologous blood or marrow transplantation. Biol Blood Marrow Transplant 2001;7(5):279–83.

[72] Chang AE, Steinberg SM, Culnane M, et al. Functional and psychosocial effects of multimodality limb-sparing therapy in patients with soft tissue sarcomas. J Clin Oncol 1989;7(9): 1217–28.

[73] Sugarbaker P, Barofsky I, Rosenberg S, et al. Quality of life assessment of patients in extremity sarcoma clinical trials. Surgery 1982;91(1):17–23.

[74] Gelfand MM. Sexuality among older women. J Womens Health Gend Based Med 2000; 9(1):15–20.

[75] Gentili A, Mulligan T. Sexual dysfunction in older adults. Clin Geriatr Med 1998;14(2): 383–93.

[76] Kandeel FR, Koussa VK, Swerdloff RS. Male sexual function and its disorders: physiology, pathophysiology, clinical investigation, and treatment. Endocr Rev 2001;22(3): 342–88.

[77] Weinrich JD. Biological research on sexual orientation: a critique of the critics. J Homosex 1995;28(1–2):197–213.

[78] Bruner DW. Maintenance of body image and sexual function. In: Watkins Bruner D, Higgs-Moore G, Haas M, editors. Outcomes in radiation therapy: multidisciplinary management. Boston: Jones and Bartlett; 2001.

[79] Gold EB, Sternfeld B, Kelsey JL, et al. Relation of demographic and lifestyle factors to symptoms in a multi-racial/ethnic population of women 40–55 years of age. Am J Epidemiol 2000;152(5):463–73.

[80] Wilson B. The effect of drugs on male sexual function and fertility. Nurse Pract 1991;16(9):12–24.

[81] Talcott JA, Manola J, Clark JA, et al. Time course and predictors of symptoms after primary prostate cancer therapy. J Clin Oncol 2003;21(21):3979–86.

[82] Basar MM, Atan A, Tekogan UY. New concept parameters of RigiScan in differentiation of vascular erectile dysfunction: is it a useful test? Int J Urol 2001;8(12):686–91.

[83] Golubinski AJ, Sikorski A. Usefulness of power doppler ultrasonography in evaluating erectile dysfunction. BJU Int 2002;89(7):779–82.

[84] Gontero P, Fontana F, Bagnasacco A, et al. Is there an optimal time for intracavernous prostaglandin E1 rehabilitation following nerve sparing radical prostatectomy? Results from a hemodynamic prospective study. J Urol 2003;169(6):2166–9.

[85] Gontero P, Fontana F, Zitella A, et al. A prospective evaluation of efficacy and compliance with a multistep treatment approach for erectile dysfunction in patients after non-nerve sparing radical prostatectomy. BJU Int 2005;95(3):359–65.

[86] Padma-Nathan H, McCullough A, Forest C. Erectile dysfunction secondary to nerve-sparing radical retropubic prostatectomy: comparative phosphodiesterase-5 inhibitor efficacy for therapy and novel prevention strategies. Curr Urol Rep 2004;5(6):467–71.

[87] Raina R, Agarwal A, Ausmundson S, et al. Early use of vacuum constriction device following radical prostatectomy facilitates early sexual activity and potentially earlier return of erectile function. Int J Impot Res 2006;18(1):77–81.

[88] Stephenson RA, Mori M, Hsieh YC, et al. Treatment of erectile dysfunction following therapy for clinically localized prostate cancer: patient reported use and outcomes from the Surveillance, Epidemiology, and End Results Prostate Cancer Outcomes Study. J Urol 2005;174(2):646–50.

[89] Gresser U, Gleiter CH. Erectile dysfunction: comparison of efficacy and side effects of the PDE-5 inhibitors sildenafil, vardenafil and tadalafil–review of the literature. Eur J Med Res 2002;7(10):435–46.

[90] Kedia S, Zippe CD, Agarwal A, et al. Treatment of erectile dysfunction with sildenafil citrate (Viagra) after radiation therapy for prostate cancer. Urology 1999;54(2):308–12.

[91] Merrick GS, Butler WM, Lief JH, et al. Efficacy of sildenafil citrate in prostate brachytherapy patients with erectile dysfunction. Urology 1999;53(6):1112–6.

[92] Weber DC, Bieri S, Kurtz JM, et al. Prospective pilot study of sildenafil for treatment of postradiotherapy erectile dysfunction in patients with prostate cancer. J Clin Oncol 1999;17(11):3444–9.

[93] Zelefsky MJ, McKee AB, Lee H, et al. Efficacy of oral sildenafil in patients with erectile dysfunction after radiotherapy for carcinoma of the prostate. Urology 1999;53(4):775–8.

[94] Incrocci L, Koper PC, Hop WC, et al. Sildenafil citrate (Viagra) and erectile dysfunction following external beam radiotherapy for prostate cancer: a randomized, double-blind, placebo-controlled, cross-over study. Int J Radiat Oncol Biol Phys 2001;51(5):1190–5.

[95] Doggrell SA. Comparison of clinical trials with sildenafil, vardenafil and tadalafil in erectile dysfunction. Expert Opin Pharmacother 2005;6(1):75–84.

[96] McCullough AR. Four-year review of sildenafil citrate. Rev Urol 2002;4(Suppl 3):S26–38.

[97] Brock G, Nehra A, Lipshultz LI, et al. Safety and efficacy of vardenafil for the treatment of men with erectile dysfunction after radical retropubic prostatectomy. J Urol 2003;170(4 Pt 1):1278–83.

[98] Nehra A, Grantmyre J, Nadel A, et al. Vardenafil improved patient satisfaction with erectile hardness, orgasmic function and sexual experience in men with erectile dysfunction following nerve sparing radical prostatectomy. J Urol 2005;173(6):2067–71.

[99] Stroberg P, Murphy A, Costigan T. Switching patients with erectile dysfunction from sildenafil citrate to tadalafil: results of a European multicenter, open-label study of patient preference. Clin Ther 2003;25(11):2724–37.

[100] Costa P, Buvat J, Holmes S, et al. Predictors of tadalafil efficacy in men with erectile dysfunction: the SURE study comparing two dosing regimens. J Sex Med 2006;3(3): 1190–5.

[101] Montorsi F, Nathan HP, McCullough A, et al. Tadalafil in the treatment of erectile dysfunction following bilateral nerve sparing radical retropubic prostatectomy: a randomized, double-blind, placebo controlled trial. J Urol 2004;172(3):1036–41.

[102] Incrocci L, Slagter C, Slob AK, et al. A randomized, double-blind, placebo-controlled, cross-over study to assess the efficacy of tadalafil (Cialis) in the treatment of erectile dysfunction following three-dimensional conformal external-beam radiotherapy for prostatic carcinoma. Int J Radiat Oncol Biol Phys 2006;66(2):439–44.

[103] Van Basten JP, Van Driel MF, Jonker-Pool G, et al. Sexual functioning in testosterone-supplemented patients treated for bilateral testicular cancer. Br J Urol 1997;79: 461–7.

[104] Montague DK, Barada JH, Belker AM, et al. Clinical guidelines panel on erectile dysfunction: summary report on the treatment of organic erectile dysfunction. J Urol 1996;156(6): 2007–11.

[105] Kava BR. Advances in the management of post-radical prostatectomy erectile dysfunction: treatment strategies when PDE-5 inhibitors don't work. Rev Urol 2005;26(6): 757–60.

[106] Costabile RA, Spevak M. Cancer and male factor infertility. Oncology 1998;12(4):565, 557–62.

[107] Raina R, Agarwal A, Ausmundson S, et al. Long-term efficacy and compliance of MUSE for erectile dysfunction following radical prostatectomy: SHIM (IIEF-5) analysis. Int J Impot Res 2005;17(1):86–90.

[108] Bosshardt RJ, Farwerk R, Sikora R, et al. Objective measurement of the effectiveness, therapeutic success and dynamic mechanisms of the vacuum device. Br J Urol 1995;75(6): 786–91.

[109] Dubocq FM, Bianco FJ Jr, Maralani SJ, et al. Outcome analysis of penile implant surgery after external beam radiation for prostate cancer. J Urol 1997;158(5):1787–90.

[110] Chye PH. Traditional Asian folklore medicines in sexual health. Indian Journal of Urology [serial online] 2006;22:241–5.

[111] Morales A. Yohimbine in erectile dysfunction: the facts. Int J Impot Res 2000;12(Suppl 1): S70–4.

[112] Guay AT, Spark RF, Jacobson J, et al. Yohimbine treatment of organic erectile dysfunction in a dose-escalation trial. Int J Impot Res 2002;14(1):25–31.

[113] Lebret T, Herve JM, Gorny P, et al. Efficacy and safety of a novel combination of L-arginine glutamate and yohimbine hydrochloride: a new oral therapy for erectile dysfunction. Eur Urol 2001;91(3):215–43.

[114] Chen J, Wollman Y, Chernichovsky T, et al. Effects of oral administration of high-dose nitric oxide donor L-arginine in men with organic erectile dysfunction: results of a double-blind, randomized, placebo-controlled study. BJU Int 1999;83(3):269–73.

[115] Murphy LL, Lee TJ. Ginseng, sex behavior, and nitric oxide. Ann N Y Acad Sci 2002;962: 372–7.

[116] Hong B, Ji YH, Hong JH, et al. A double-blind crossover study evaluating the efficacy of Korean red ginseng in patients with erectile dysfunction: a preliminary report. J Urol 2002; 168(5):2070–3.

[117] Yaman LS, Kilic S, Sarica K, et al. The place of acupuncture in the management of psychogenic impotence. Eur Urol 1994;26(1):52–5.

[118] Kho HG, Sweep CG, Chen X, et al. The use of acupuncture in the treatment of erectile dysfunction. Int J Impot Res 1999;11(1):41–6.

[119] Neese LE, Schover LR, Klein EA, et al. Finding help for sexual problems after prostate cancer treatment: a phone survey of men's and women's perspectives. Psychooncology 2003;12(5):463–73.

[120] Titta M, Tavolini IM, Moro FD, et al. Sexual counseling improved erectile rehabilitation after non-nerve-sparing radical retropubic prostatectomy or cystectomy–results of a randomized prospective study. J Sex Med 2006;3(2):267–73.

[121] Canada AL, Neese LE, Sui D, et al. Pilot intervention to enhance sexual rehabilitation for couples after treatment for localized prostate carcinoma. Cancer 2005;104(12): 2689–700.

ELSEVIER
SAUNDERS

Nurs Clin N Am 42 (2007) 581–592

NURSING
CLINICS
OF NORTH AMERICA

The Impact of Diabetes Mellitus on Female Sexual Well-Being

Cindy Grandjean, PhD, CANP/GNP*,
Barbara Moran, PhD, CNM, FACCE

The Catholic University of America, Washington, DC, USA

According to the American Diabetes Association, 7% of Americans (20.8 million) have been diagnosed with diabetes mellitus [1]. Researchers have reported that a woman's risk for developing diabetes sometime during her life has reached "epidemic proportions in the U.S.," particularly for minority women [2]. It has been estimated that diabetes impacts close to 10 million American women, and that approximately 9% of all women aged 20 years or older have diabetes [3]. The incidence of diabetes is two to four times higher for African American, Hispanic/Latino, American Indian and Asian/Pacific Islander women, when compared with Caucasian women [1].

Diabetes has a significantly detrimental effect on many body systems, including the renal, nervous, and cardiovascular systems [4]. As a result of the impact of diabetes on these systems, individuals with diabetes suffer from various medical and psychologic problems. A growing number of researchers are beginning to explore the impact these medical and psychologic complications have on sexual well-being.

Researchers have identified that sexual dysfunction in diabetic men has been linked to vascular alterations, endocrine abnormalities, psychologic problems, and neurologic deficits [5]. Although less evidence exists on the relationship among diabetes, the female genitourinary system, and sexual dysfunction in women, sexual dysfunction has been identified as a prevalent problem in women, and some evidence indicates that diabetes increases the risk for sexual dysfunction in this population [6]. More specifically, Doruk and colleagues [7] evaluated risk factors associated with sexual dysfunction in a cohort of 127 married women: 21 women with type 1 diabetes, 50 women with type 2 diabetes, and 56 healthy women. Participants were given a questionnaire that asked about sexual desire, arousal, lubrication, orgasm,

---

* Corresponding author.
  E-mail address: grandjean@cua.edu (C. Grandjean).

0029-6465/07/$ - see front matter © 2007 Elsevier Inc. All rights reserved.
doi:10.1016/j.cnur.2007.08.004   *nursing.theclinics.com*

pain, and satisfaction. Seventy-one percent of the group with type 1 diabetes reported sexual dysfunction. The prevalence of sexual dysfunction in the type 2 diabetic group and control group was 42% and 37%, respectively.

As long ago as 1974, the World Health Organization recognized that human sexuality is an important element of an individual's health and well-being [8]. Therefore, it is vital that clinicians address the issue of sexuality with their female diabetic patients. This article provides a brief review of the literature, followed by a discussion addressing the proper approach for sexual dysfunction screening. Finally, this article considers some of the current and future treatment modalities that can be used to enhance sexual functioning in female diabetics with impaired sexual function.

Review of the literature

In the past, the impact of diabetes on sexuality was often overlooked by scientists. In fact, even discussing the topic of sexuality was deemed "taboo" before 1940 and therefore, it was not addressed in the literature. The philosophy before the 1940s has been characterized as, "If you don't ask about it, it doesn't exist" [6]. After this time frame, the medical community started to recognize the impact of diabetes on sexuality, but only as it related to men. It wasn't until 1971 that researchers conducted one of the first studies that looked at the sexual functioning of women with diabetes mellitus. In his study, Kolodny [9] reported that 35% of the diabetes mellitus women identified an inability to achieve an orgasm, versus 6% of nondiabetic women. This researcher linked this anorgasmia directly to diabetes mellitus.

Schreiner-Engel and colleagues [10] also investigated diabetes and female sexuality by comparing the cognitive, psychologic, interpersonal, and sexual dimensions of 50 women with diabetes to 50 matched controls. In this study, although diabetic women had relatively little impairment in their sexual responses, their sexual desire was significantly lower. A decrease in lubrication was reported, although its adequacy for coitus was not perceived differently by the two groups.

More recently, Enzlin and colleagues [11] completed an investigation on sexual dysfunction in healthy women and in those with type 1 diabetes mellitus. These researchers set out to address some of the limitations of previous studies by using a larger sample size (120 women) with just type 1 diabetics and a control group. The objectives of this research were to examine the prevalence of sexual problems in women with type 1 diabetes mellitus and to evaluate the influence of somatic complaints related to diabetes on female sexuality. Women in this study were given a questionnaire with items that assessed sexual function and items that addressed whether this dysfunction caused "marked personal distress or interpersonal difficulty." Participants completed questions relating to depression and the quality of their marital relations. The diabetic women completed inventories relating to their disease. The results from this study were that the type 1 diabetic women reported significantly more sexual dysfunction, and that these problems are often related to sexual arousal. When compared with the control group (6%), the diabetic women (14%) reported a statistically significant difference for decreased vaginal lubrication. The diabetic women also reported more frequent problems with sexual desire, orgasm, and dyspareunia, although these findings were not statistically significant. The investigators of this study concluded that the diabetic women appeared to be more at risk for sexual dysfunction, specifically relating to the arousal phase, and psychologic factors such as depression and disease acceptance.

Enzlin and his colleagues [12] expanded on this study by investigating whether diabetic women are at higher risk for sexual dysfunction, just as diabetic men are. This descriptive study of 240 adult patients who had type 1 diabetes found that the prevalence rates of sexual dysfunction in diabetic men and diabetic women were 22% and 27%, respectively. Although the researchers found that women with diabetes have the same risk for sexual dysfunction as men with diabetes, this study suggested that "in men with diabetes, sexual dysfunction is related to somatic and psychological factors, whereas in women with diabetes, psychological factors are more predominant."

Rutherford and Collier [5] conducted a comprehensive review of the literature as it pertained to the incidence and etiology of sexual dysfunction among diabetic women. These researchers particularly focused on the factors (ie, vascular disease, endocrine problems, and psychologic problems) that have been linked with diabetic male sexual dysfunction. From their literature search, these investigators found some evidence that an alteration in blood supply secondary to diabetes mellitus may influence sexual outcomes in women. Blood flow to the female genitalia serves several purposes in sexual function. In preparation for coitus, during the arousal stage, the perivaginal tissues become vasocongested. This vasogestion serves to enhance clitoral stimulation by way of clitoral tumescence. Without an adequate supply of blood to the vaginal structures, the introitus atrophies. Atrophic changes and decreased lubrication have been associated with dyspareunia and a decreased sensation of the clitoris. Rutherford and Collier [5] also speculated that vasocongestion may be compromised by a decrease in nitric oxide levels. They reported that a possible complication of diabetes is decreased levels of nitric oxide due to vascular disease and that this substance plays an important role in penile tumescence. Rutherford and Collier's review focused on the impact of hormonal alterations in diabetic woman as they related to sexual drive. From this analysis, they concluded that "vascular pathology and neuropathy in conjunction with elevated serum androgens particularly in women with type 2 diabetes is likely to have an adverse effect on sexuality and sexual function."

Several studies have identified a possible connection between psychologic factors and sexual functioning in diabetic women. Sexual dysfunction is associated with a lower overall quality of marital relations and more depressive symptoms in diabetic women [13]. Depression may have an effect on sexual function and reports indicate that depression is three times more common among individuals with diabetes than the general population [14]. It is often difficult to determine whether diabetes or depression is causing the sexual dysfunction. LeMone [15] reported that other problems affecting women's sexuality were fatigue, changes in premenstrual blood, glucose control, vaginitis, decreased sexual desire, decreased vaginal lubrication, and an increased time to reach orgasm. In another qualitative study, Sarkadi and Rosenqvist [16] identified guilt and embarrassment regarding their diabetes, vaginal dryness, pain during intercourse, and decreased desire as affecting sexual functioning.

Historically, research on the impact of diabetes on sexuality in women has not been conducted. Recently, researchers found that vascular pathology is likely to have an adverse effect on sexuality and sexual function. Studies have confirmed that diabetes decreases vaginal lubrication, decreases sexual desire and orgasm, and increases dysypareunia. Additionally, it has been found that psychological factors such as depression and fatigue are predominant issues in diabetic women.

Screening for sexual well-being

The health assessment and screening of diabetic women need to be approached in a holistic, nonjudgmental manner, taking into consideration age and cultural, religious, and educational factors. In addition to current and past medical problems, including chronic illness, it is important to obtain a detailed obstetric and gynecologic history of the patient. For example, women should be asked specifically about any gynecologic or pelvic surgeries, such as a hysterectomy or fallopian tube surgeries, because these may possibly influence sexual response. "It is possible that decreased vasocongestion and lack of uterine contractions with orgasm could alter a woman's sexual response" [17]. Endometriosis could be the cause of dyspareunia. A vaginal discharge or irritation could indicate an infection. If the woman is peri- or postmenopausal, decreasing estrogen levels may result in decreased vaginal lubrication, causing pain and loss of desire.

Practitioners need to review the medications the patients are taking because some medications could have an impact on sexual functioning. For example, medications that alter blood flow, such as an antihypertensive drug, and medications that dry mucous membranes, such as an antihistamine, may influence sexual functioning. Other drugs that may influence sexual function include antidepressants, antipsychotics, narcotics, oral contraceptives, and drugs like cocaine and marijuana. Alcohol can also alter the sexual response [18].

Identifying any psychiatric disorders, such as depression, anxiety, low self-esteem, or alcohol abuse, is important in the assessment of the diabetic woman because, as stated earlier, untreated depression or anxiety can inhibit a woman's ability to engage in the sexual experience, which will result in decrease lubrication and pain with intercourse [19].

Finally, assessing for intimate partner violence is essential in all assessments of women. The following simple questions should be asked: "Within the last year, have you been hit, slapped, kicked, or otherwise physically hurt by someone?" and "Within the last year, has anyone forced you to have sexual activities?" [19].

Because many women are reluctant to discuss sexual issues, asking women with diabetes about their sexual concerns as a routine part of assessment will give them a chance to "discuss both sexual and social intimacy concerns related to their diabetes" [16]. Taking a sexual assessment may take the practitioner longer than other types of assessments "in part because the emotional experience of sexual function/dysfunction is as relevant as the dysfunction per se" [20].

Initial assessment can be achieved by asking a couple of open-ended questions, such as

- Are you having any sexual difficulty at this time?
- Do you have any sexual concerns or problems?
- Some of my patients complain of pain with sex. Has this happened to you?

If the practitioner receives a positive response to these questions, then he/she should try to identify the specific concerns [20]:

1. Ask the patient to describe the problem in her own words. This question will help clarify the issue.
2. Determine the duration of the problem to assess whether the problem is generalized or situational.
3. Determine the context of the sexual problem. This assessment will include the expectations of, and communication between, the partners, and the patient's relationship with her partner.
4. Determine the rest of the sexual response. Does she experiencing a decrease in arousal and desire?
5. Assess reaction by inquiring how each partner has reacted to the problem.
6. Ask the patient whether she has undertaken any previous treatment or self-help.

At the end of the history and physical, women may need to be referred for psychologic counseling or sex therapy, as indicated.

Treatment modalities

To provide effective treatment modalities for female sexual dysfunction, practitioners must conduct a thorough history and physical. As mentioned previously, a complete examination should include a sexual history to help identify specific issues relating to sexual dysfunction. The literature indicates that diabetic women may be at higher risk for sexual dysfunction because of vaginal dryness, dyspareunia, decreased arousal or desire, and psychologic factors. Treatment modalities are discussed for each of these specific problems.

Vaginal dryness

Vaginal dryness is a medical complaint that is often minimized or overlooked by patients and practitioners in order to address more "pressing" problems [21]. As indicated in the literature, decreased vaginal lubrication among diabetic women is a common complaint and, if not addressed, can lead to dyspareunia, urinary symptoms, and vaginal infections [6]. To treat this problem effectively, practitioners need to assess for contributing factors, such as use of vaginal products. Patients should be advised to avoid using douches, chemicals, strong soaps, and perfumes in the vagina because they may not only irritate the vaginal tissues but may also create an imbalance in the environment of the vagina, which may lead to bacterial and yeast infections [22].

Patients may try many over-the-counter remedies to help alleviate vaginal dryness. Practitioners should be specific about recommendations for vaginal lubricants or vaginal moisturizers because oil-based lubrications, such as mineral oil and baby oil, may threaten the integrity of latex condoms and diaphragms [23]. Generally, lubricants are considered temporary measures to relieve vaginal dryness during intercourse. Their formulations are a combination of protectants and thickening agents in a water-soluble base. Lubricants can be applied frequently and, because their action is limited in duration, they require reapplication before sexual activity. Vaginal moisturizers, such as Replens, which is meant to be used on a more regular basis, claim to moisturize the vagina and provide more than transient lubrication. They are promoted as providing long-term relief of vaginal dryness, rather than being just sexual aids. Table 1 [24] provides a list of some over-the-counter products recommended for treatment of vaginal dryness.

Health care providers should also assess a women's pleasuring (foreplay) pattern, because more time and stimulation are often necessary for adequate lubrication of vaginal and clitoral tissues. Therefore, women should be advised to elongate the time spent during foreplay with use of erotic material or a vibrator to enhance stimulation.

Another essential factor for proper vaginal lubrication is adequate amounts of estrogen. In fact, the American College of Obstetricians and Gynecologists has stated that "vaginal estrogen cream, the vaginal ring and even low doses of estrogen in the form of pills or patches can help relieve vaginal dryness and improve lubrication" [25]. Practitioners may consider the initiation of hormone replacement therapy or estrogen replacement therapy in women who are perimenopausal, menopausal, status post-hysterectomy, or who have received treatment for certain types of cancer. It is

Table 1
Over-the-counter products recommended for treatment of vaginal dryness

	Specific characteristics	Instructions for patient
Vaginal lubricants		
K-Y Jelly	Inexpensive	Recommended for episodic use
	Water soluble	with sexual intercourse
Astroglide	Water soluble, pH balanced,	May impede sperm motility,
	water based, and	thereby impacting female
	petroleum free	fertility
	Tubes prepackaged in	May increase the risk of
	single-dose syringes	condom slippage during
Lubrin	Water soluble and nonstaining	vaginal sex
	Can be applied well before	(pharmacotherapy) [27]
	intercourse and liquefies	
	only inside the body	
	Manufactured in a pessary	
	form	
Vaginal moisturizers		
Replens	Bioadhesive ingredient,	Forms moist coating on the
	polycarbophil polymer,	surface of vaginal cells
	attaches to mucin and	Application every 3 d
	epithelial cells on the	Lowers vaginal pH through its
	vaginal wall through	weak acidity (pH 2.8) and
	anionic binding.	buffering capacity
	Polycarbophil carries up	May result in vaginal residue
	to 60 times its weight in	[24]
	water and holds water in	May impede sperm motility,
	place against the vaginal	thereby impacting female
	epithelial surface until it	fertility
	is sloughed off, typically	
	after 24 hours or more	
Moist Again Vaginal	Specifically formulated to	
Moisturizing Gel	provide long-lasting relief	
	of vaginal dryness and can	
	be used daily	
	Fragrance and irritant free and	
	does not contain petroleum	
	or mineral oil, so it is safe to	
	use with latex condoms	

vital that providers work together with their female patients to decide whether the benefits of using hormone or estrogen therapy for relief of vaginal dryness and vaginal pain are worth the risk.

Dyspareunia

Dyspareunia may be associated with certain pathologic conditions of the genital structures. Therefore, practitioners need to identify and treat specific problems associated with dyspareunia, such as herpetic lesions, vaginal infections, and allergic reactions [23]. For many women with dyspareunia, the examination reveals no obvious pathology, but instead, the practitioner notes changes associated with urogenital atrophy. This condition is most frequently seen in women with low estrogen levels, which result in flattening of rugations, vaginal thinning, and decreased lubrication [23].

This problem responds well to estrogen therapy because estrogen restores vaginal elasticity and thickening by increasing vaginal blood flow, generally within 6 weeks of therapy. Topical estrogen therapies applied to the outer third of the vagina optimizes outcomes [26]. Another option to consider may be the estrogen ring, which is inserted every 3 months into the upper third of the vagina. This ring releases a more continuous dose of estrogen but it has very little systemic absorption; therefore, it may not require progesterone opposition [27]. Long-term use of topical estrogen therapy does require administration of progesterone opposition. See Table 2 for list of topical and vaginal estrogen products.

Other therapies that may minimize dyspareunia are a warm bath before intercourse, topical lidocaine, biofeedback, and avoidance of sexual positions that exacerbate the discomfort [26]. Vaginal lubricants or moisturizers may be used, with or without estrogen therapies, to address vaginal friction secondary to vaginal dryness. Also, practitioners may teach women pelvic exercises (ie, Kegel exercises) for vaginal muscle relaxation. Progressive muscle relaxation can be taught during an instructional examination by having the patient alternate contracting and relaxing the pelvic muscles around the examiner's finger [28].

Sexual arousal and desire issues

When treating a woman with sexual arousal difficulties, practitioners must keep in mind that sexual desire depends on mood, motivation to sexual intimacy, and hormonal factors [12]. The most common hormonally related problem associated with diminished sexual arousal is estrogen because sexual arousal is influenced by levels of this chemical. Women experiencing estrogen deficiencies at menopause are often impacted by changes in vaginal structure and function. These changes can result in delayed arousal.

Another hormonal deficiency that may impact sexual arousal and desire is testosterone. Testosterone appears to have a direct impact on female sexual arousal and sexual desire [29]. Treatment with testosterone is

Table 2
Topical and vaginal estrogen products

Vaginal creams	Estrace	0.1% estradiol
	Ogen	1.5 mg/estropipate
	Premarin	0.625 mg/g natural conjugated estrogen
Vaginal rings	Femring	0.05, 0.1 mg/d estradiol acetate
	Estring	2 mg 17 beta-estradiol
	Menoring	0.05, 0.1 mg/d estradiol acetate

controversial because findings in the literature have been mixed. Some studies have found that androgen therapy improves libido, sexual arousal, and frequency of sexual fantasies [29,30], whereas others have reported no significant benefits [31,32]. The most significant benefits of androgen therapy have been noted among women who have undergone bilateral oophorectomy and subsequently developed a decrease in sexual libido.

Along with these inconclusive findings, testosterone therapy has been associated with potential adverse effects such as a decline in serum high density lipoprotein cholesterol, clitorimegaly, and voice deepening [33]. Although rare, testosterone therapy has also been associated with hepatocellular damage.

Testosterone can be administered by way of injection, creams, gels, tablets, pellets, and transdermally. No guidelines for testosterone replacement therapy for women with disorders of desire and no consensus of "normal" or "therapeutic" levels of testosterone therapy exist [28]. Before initiating testosterone treatment, physicians should discuss the potential and theoretic risks, and the individual risk and benefit assessment, with the patient. In general, patients who have, or have had, breast cancer, uncontrolled hyperlipidemia, liver disease, acne, or hirsutism should not receive testosterone therapy. The potential cardiovascular side effects of long-term testosterone use may be of more concern for practitioners who are treating sexual dysfunction in diabetic women [34]. The administration of estrogen with testosterone (ie, Estratest or Estratest HS) has been shown to negate the effects of testosterone on lipoproteins.

Psychosocial issues

Sexual well-being is a function of healthy relationships. Positive sexual activity requires honest communication; therefore, partners should be encouraged to discuss this topic openly. Specifically, partners should be discussing such things as: what specific sexual problems may be present; what stimulates or diminishes sexual desire; and what enhances each other's self-image. Also, regular sexual activity actually has been shown to promote sexual well-being, in that sexual activity helps maintain vaginal pH, Po_2, and mucosal health [35]. Practitioners should consider referring couples for sexual counseling when appropriate [35].

Diabetic women may be at increased risk for depression. Primary care providers may need to address this issue with the initiation of medication. If so, one should be aware that some antidepressants may produce sexual side effects.

Therapies for the future

Researchers are exploring the impact of other medications and products to address female sexual dysfunction. Sildenafil is a medication that is currently being tested for its effectiveness in addressing female sexual arousal disorders. Although the preliminary findings are mixed, some evidence indicates that sildenafil improves arousal, sexual enjoyment, and dyspareunia in type 1 diabetic women [36,37]. Tibolone is another medication that may be used by practitioners in the near future to address sexual arousal disorders in women. Some evidence indicates that tibolone increases vaginal lubrication, arousability, and sexual desire in postmenopausal women [38].

Scientists have also developed a new mechanical product intended to increase genital blood flow. This clitoral suction devise, available in United States, uses suction or negative pressure to increase vasocongestion and engorge the clitoris and paraclitoral tissues for enhanced arousal and orgasm. This clitoral pump, known as the Eros-Clitoral Therapy Device, is only available with a prescription [39].

Summary

For women, the risk for developing diabetes mellitus is reaching epidemic levels. As a result of the impact of diabetes on multiple body systems, women may suffer from medical and psychologic problems, including sexual dysfunction. In all probability, it is a combination of factors that influences the sexual response of diabetic women. It is difficult to separate sexual response from the many emotional and other contributing factors that may influence a relationship. Therefore, it is vital that clinicians address the issue of sexuality with their female diabetic patients. Providers must incorporate sexual screening in women with diabetes, along with thorough physical examinations, to identify and treat this problem effectively. Also, researchers need to continue to explore the relationship between diabetes and sexual dysfunction in women.

References

[1] All about diabetes. American Diabetes Association Web site. Available at: www.diabetes. org/about-diabetes.jsp. Accessed February 9, 2007.
[2] Wider J. Surge in diabetes among women and minorities. Society for Women's Health Research Website. Available at: http://www.womenshealthresearch.org/site/News2? page=NewsArticle&;id=5356&news_iv_ctrl=0&abbr=press_. Accessed February 9, 2007.
[3] National Diabetes Statistics Web site. Available at: www.diabetes.niddk.nih.gov/dm/pubs/ statistics. Accessed Feb 9, 2007.
[4] DCCT Research Group. The effect of intensive treatment of diabetes on the development and progression of long-term complications. N Engl J Med 1993;329:977–86.
[5] Rutherford D, Collier A. Sexual dysfunction in women with diabetes mellitus. Gynecol Endocrinol 2005;21:189–92.
[6] Enzlin P, et al. Diabetes and female sexual functioning: a state-of-the-art. Diabetes Spectrum 2003;16:256–9.
[7] Doruk H, Akbay E, Cayan S, et al. Effect of diabetes mellitus on female sexual function and risk factors. Archives of Andrology 2005;51:1–6.

[8] Education & treatment in human sexuality: the training of health professionals. WHO. Available at: www2.hu-berlin.die/sexology/GESUND/ARCHIV/CHRO7.htm. Accessed June 9, 2007.

[9] Kolodny RC. Sexual dysfunction in diabetic females. Diabetes 1971;20:557–9.

[10] Schreiner-Engel P, Schiavi R, Vietorisz D, et al. Diabetes and female sexuality: a comparative study of women in relationships. J Sex Marital Ther 1985;11:165–75.

[11] Enzlin P, Chantal M, Van den Bruel A. Sexual dysfunction in women with type 1 diabetes: a controlled study. Diabetes Care 2002;25:672–7.

[12] Enzlin P, Mathieu C, Van den Bruel A, et al. Prevalence and predictors of sexual dysfunction in patients with type 1 diabetes mellitus. Diabetes Care 2003;26:409–14.

[13] Morano S. Pathophysiology of diabetic sexual dysfunction. J Endocrinol Invest 2003;26: 65–9.

[14] Diabetes and female sexuality, Medihealth DME Web site. Available at: www. medihealthdme.com/education/diabetes_femalesex.htm. Accessed February 9, 2007.

[15] LeMone P. The physical effects of diabetes on sexuality in women. Diabetes Educ 1996;22: 361–6.

[16] Sarkadi A, Rosenqvist U. Intimacy and women with type 2 diabetes: an exploratory study using focus group interviews. Diabetes Educ 2003;29:641–52.

[17] Seltzer V, Pearse W, editors. Women's primary health care. New York: McGraw-Hill; 2000. p. 458.

[18] Gross G. Women and sexuality. In: Curtis M, Overholt S, Hopkins M, editors. Glass' office gynecology. Philadelphia: Lippincott Williams & Wilkins; 2006. p. 560–73.

[19] McFarlane J, Parker B, Moran B. Abuse during pregnancy: a protocol for prevention and intervention. 3rd edition. New York: March of Dimes; 2007.

[20] Basson R. Introduction to special issue on women's sexuality and outline of assessment of sexual problems. Menopause 2004;11:709–13.

[21] Seibel M. Four steps to non-hormonal treatment of vaginal dryness. Available at: http://www.ourgyn.com/article. Accessed February 15, 2007.

[22] Iannacchione MA. The vagina dialogues: do you douche? Am J Nurs 2004;104:40–5.

[23] Hatcher R, Trussel J, Stewart F. Contraceptive technology. New York: Ardent Media; 2004.

[24] Caswell M, Kane M. Comparison of the moisturization efficacy of two vaginal moisturizers: pectin versus polycarbophil technologies. J Cosmet Sci 2002;53:81–7.

[25] Frequently asked questions about hormone therapy: new recommendations based on ACOG's Task Force report on HT. American College of Obstetricians and Gynecologists. Available at: www.acog.org/from_home/publications/press_releases/nr10-01-04.cfm. Accessed June 9, 2007.

[26] Striar S, Bartlik B. Stimulation of the libido: the use of erotica in sex therapy. Psychiatr Ann 1999;29:60–2.

[27] Willhite L, O'Connell M. Urogenital atrophy: prevention and treatment. Pharmacotherapy 2001;21(4):464–80.

[28] Phillips N. Female sexual dysfunction: evaluation and treatment. Am Fam Physician 2000; 62:127–36, 141–2.

[29] Davis SR, Burger HG. Clinical review 82: androgens and the postmenopausal woman. J Clin Endocrinol Metab 1996;81:2759–63.

[30] Sherwin BB, Gelfand MM, Brender W. Androgen enhances sexual motivation in females: a prospective, crossover study of sex steroid administration in the surgical menopause. Psychosom Med 1985;47:339–51.

[31] Myers LS, Dixen J, Morrissette D, et al. Effects of estrogen, androgen, and progestin on sexual psychophysiology and behavior in postmenopausal women. J Clin Endocrinol Metab 1990;70:1124–31.

[32] Dennerstein L, Dudley EC, Hopper JL, et al. Sexuality, hormones and the menopausal transition. Maturitas 1997;26:83–93.

[33] Slayden SM. Risks of menopausal androgen supplementation. Semin Reprod Endocrinol 1998;16:145–52.
[34] Lemecke D, Pattison J, Marshall L, et al. Current care of women: diagnosis & treatment. New York: Lan/McGraw-Hill; 2004.
[35] Altman A. Etiology and diagnosis of sexual dysfunction in women. Up-To-Date. Available at: http://www.patients.uptodate.com. Accessed February 12, 2007.
[36] Caruso S, Rugolo S, Agnello C, et al. Sildenafil improves sexual functioning in premenopausal women with type 1 diabetes who are affected by sexual arousal disorder: a double-blind, crossover, placebo-controlled pilot study. Fertil Steril 2006;85:1496–501.
[37] Caruso S, Rugolo S, Mirabella D, et al. Changes in clitoral blood flow in premenopausal women affected by type 1 diabetes after signle100-mg administration of sildenafil. Urology 2006;68:161–5.
[38] Laan E, Van Lunsen RH, Everaerd W. The effects of tibolone on vaginal blood flow, sexual desire and arousability in postmenopausal women. Climacteric 2001;4:28–41.
[39] Wilson SK, Delk JR, Billups KL. Treating symptoms of female sexual arousal disorder with the Eros-Clitoral Therapy Device. J Gend Specif Med 2001;4:54–8.

ELSEVIER
SAUNDERS

NURSING
CLINICS
OF NORTH AMERICA

Nurs Clin N Am 42 (2007) 593–603

Cardiac Disease and Sexuality: Implications for Research and Practice

Sonya R. Hardin, RN, PhD, CCRN

School of Nursing, Room 444F, College of Health and Human Services, University of North Carolina at Charlotte, 9201 University City Boulevard, Charlotte, NC 28223, USA

Popular culture has portrayed cardiovascular disease in movies, such as *As Good as it Gets* with Jack Nicholson as a survivor of a myocardial infarction (MI). Nicholson's character was characterized as being driven by his sexual prowess and the issues around his ability to return to an active sexual performance state. Movies such as this have brought to the forefront the issues of sexuality and cardiovascular disease (CVD). The public's understanding of cardiovascular disease and its relationship to sexuality would lead one to believe that there exists a narrow view of sexuality as an act that is limited when one has cardiovascular disease. While the movie does highlight that sex is a contributor to one's quality of life, research has shown a 2.1% risk of myocardial infarction 1 hour post sexual intercourse [1]. Nevertheless, in the minds of the public, cardiovascular disease and sexuality are often perceived to be noncoexistent.

Given that cardiovascular disease is the leading cause of illness and death in the United States, and that 40% of the population between the ages of 40 and 59 has cardiovascular disease, a percentage that increases to 75% between the ages of 60 and 79, with further increases noted at age 80 to be approximately 87%, understanding sexuality is paramount. Currently, an estimated one in three American adults have some form of CVD [2]. Half of these individuals are age 65 or older. One in six adults over the age of 55 will have a stroke. Hypertension is found in one out of four individuals aged 35 to 44. Approximately half of the people age 55 will have hypertension. Approximately 37.5% of men in the United States aged 45 to 55, 49% aged 55 to 65, and 63.6% over the age of 65 have hypertension [2]. Mortality related to CVD in 2004 was the underlying cause of death in one out of every 2.8 deaths in the United States. An average of one death every 36 seconds is attributable to CVD. As health care

E-mail address: srhardin@uncc.edu

providers, our focus is to reduce risk of this disease by focusing on the reduction of the three major risk factors: hypertension, smoking, and elevated total cholesterol 240 mg/dL. Yet, even with all the research focused on various interventions, protocol development, and guideline implementation, the estimated direct and indirect cost of CVD for 2007 is $431.8 billion [2].

Cardiovascular disease includes the medical diagnosis of coronary heart disease, acute coronary syndrome, angina pectoris, hypertension, heart failure, stroke, and transient ischemic attacks. With the diagnosis of CVD, lifestyle changes are recommended that are critical to managing the disease. As the disease process progresses, individuals face issues that can impact quality of life. One such issue is sexuality, which encompasses sexual behavior and sexual desire [3]. Sexual behavior can be expressed alone, with another, or with others through a variety of intimate acts that may differ given the disease process. Given that cardiovascular disease is most prominent in mid-life (40–59 years) and late life (60–79 years), sexuality should be understood as a developmental process. With maturity comes a broader understanding of sexual behavior and sexual desire that must be considered in overseeing the care of individuals with cardiovascular disease.

The purpose of this article is to discuss the physiologic effects of sexual intercourse on the heart, review the current literature on sexuality in various types of CVD, and the nurse's role in promoting and maintaining the sexual health of a patient's diagnoses with CVD. The impacts of cardiovascular symptoms, such as fatigue, depression, shortness of breath, chest pain, emotional stress, and overactive bladder disease or urinary incontinence on sexuality are also discussed.

Physiologic effects of sexual intercourse on the heart

Historically, sexual intercourse and sexual desire among individuals with a cardiac history have been viewed as being associated with increased demands on the cardiovascular system, regardless of sexual orientation. The effects of cardiovascular disease on sexuality are multiple and can impact all the phases of sexual response. In both genders, there are four stages of sexual response: excitement, plateau, orgasmic, and resolution.

The first stage of excitement results in emotional changes, vasoconstriction, and vaginal lubrication caused by vascular engorgement of the vaginal wall, an increase in heart rate, blood pressure, and respiration. In combination with vasoconstriction are mild vasocongestion within the clitoris and a slight swelling in the breasts; in addition, the nipples may become erect. In the male, an erection results from an increase in vasocongestion. During this first stage, the increase in blood pressure, heart rate, and respirations may increase fatigue of the late-stage CVD patient and prevent the individual from moving into the second phase.

The second stage of sexual response, called the plateau, happens when vasocongestion reaches its maximum. In both the male and female, the plateau stage includes an increase in muscle tension, heart rate, breathing rate, and blood pressure. Breathing and heart rates increase, not because of physical activity but because of stimulation from the autonomic (sympathetic) nervous system. Masters and Johnson [4] found that briefly before orgasm tachycardia, ranging in a rate of 110 to 180 beats per minute, and an increase of 40-mm to 80-mm systolic and 20-mm to 50-mm diastolic occurred. In the male, the glans (head) of the penis turns a deeper red or purplish color and a few drops of slippery fluid may be released from the urethra. In the female, the labia appear darker in color, the clitoris retracts, and small glands outside the vaginal opening secrete a mucus-like fluid. It is during this second stage of sexual response that interventions for the cardiovascular patient have been targeted, such as prophylactic nitroglycerin to prevent angina.

The third stage of sexual response is known as the orgasmic phase, which is both the most intense and short-lived stage. During orgasm in both males and females the heart rate, blood pressure, and breathing rate all reach peak levels. For the male, orgasm almost always includes ejaculation, which occurs as phase 1, emission, and phase 2, expulsion. Phase 1 is when semen is collecting in the urethral bulb and a feeling of being on the verge of ejaculation occurs. This phase last several seconds and represents a point when orgasm is about to occur. Phase 2 is expulsion, which results in rhythmic contractions of the muscles around the base of the penis and anus. Semen is propelled down the urethra because of these muscular contractions. For the female, the orgasmic phase involves rhythmic contractions of the uterus and the muscles that surround the vagina [4]. Most women require direct stimulation of the clitoris for an orgasm to occur [5]. Given the need for direct stimulation, orgasm can be reached much more easily and faster through masturbation than through intercourse. Factors influencing orgasm in both men and women include a person's mood, psychologic state, level of desire, relation to partner, drug or alcohol use, expectations, physical condition, and time since the last orgasm.

The fourth stage of sexual response is resolution, when the body returns back to its nonaroused state. During this stage the labia turn back to their normal coloration and the vagina, clitoris, and penis return to normal size and position. Following an orgasm, heart rate and blood pressure drop to normal ranges [4].

The most significant physiologic change during sexual response is in the cardiovascular system. Studies performed in the 1960s examined changes in heart rate and systolic blood pressure of healthy men during sexual intercourse in various positions (the missionary position or man-on-top, and the woman-on-top position). Findings suggested that exertion during sexual intercourse corresponds to that posed by a physical activity involving mild-to-moderate energy expenditure. Mild-to-moderate physical activity would include walking up to 5 km per hour, taking two flights of stairs, driving a car, or discussing business matters [6–8]. Research has concluded that energy expenditure during intercourse is dependent upon the sexual modality. The most energy expenditure is noted with the person who is on top during the missionary position. The next least amount of energy expended is with the person that is on the bottom during the use of the missionary position. The smallest amount of energy is expended with self-stimulation or partner stimulation [9]. The literature is lacking on the level of energy expenditure with other sexual modalities (eg, extramarital sexual activity, oral sex, or homosexual activity, among others).

Review of the current literature on sexuality in various types of cardiovascular disease

Sexual desire does not dissipate as one ages. On the contrary, research has shown that the majority of older adults believe that quality of life is enhanced with sexual activity and that sexual activity is part of a good relationship [10]. Barriers to the fulfillment of sexual desires has been associated with a lack of maintaining erections, vaginal lubrication, and desire associated with medications and chronic illness [11–13]. Chronic health problems were found to restrict sexual activity in 20% of respondents [10], which is not surprising considering that symptoms such as fatigue, depression, shortness of breath, chest pain, emotional stress, and medications, such as those used to treat depression and hypertension, can impact sexuality in chronic illness. Besides the severity of disease or medical treatment, other issues impacting sexuality are fatigue, body image, fear, and caregiving duties. Fig. 1 presents a model explicating the forces impacting sexuality in the cardiovascular patient.

The Princeton consensus panel has made recommendations on the clinical management of sexual dysfunction in cardiovascular patients, regardless of the type of heart disease being experienced [6]. Through the identification

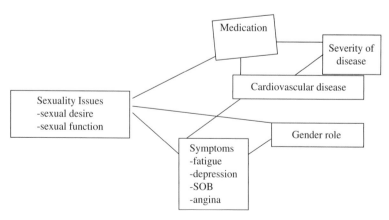

Fig. 1. Model of cardiovascular disease and sexuality.

of three categories of cardiovascular disease—low risk, intermediate risk, and high risk—clinical recommendations are made on interventions for sexual dysfunction. Those individuals in the low-risk group (stable) should be encouraged to initiate or resume sexual activity. The low-risk group should be treated for sexual dysfunction. The intermediate-risk group should receive further cardiac diagnostic examination to stratify as stable or unstable. The high-risk group (unstable) should receive cardiac treatment and become stable before the initiation or resumption of sexual activity. Typically, those in the high-risk group should be stabilized before treating any sexual dysfunction. Table 1 displays the cardiac disease by risk category.

Severity of the disease

The severity of cardiovascular disease is dependent upon the symptoms the patient experiences, which can range from angina, shortness of breath, fatigue, or low blood sugar (those with diabetes). Interventions, such as self-medication with nitroglycerin to prevent pain during sexual intercourse, or having a rest before initiation can be beneficial. However, if a couple has a mental model that their sex life is over because of the illness, they will need help in redefining their sexual relationship to include other sexual behaviors besides intercourse [14]. The severity of the disease often requires the patient and spouse to redefine roles. In situations where the male had a more active sexual role before CVD, the couple may have trouble coping with the need to change roles. Couples that have been together for many years often have established routines related to their sexual behavior and will need help in negotiating new roles [14].

Cardiovascular medications impacting sexuality

Many medications will impact sexual desire; however, most of the cardiovascular medications have the potential to impact desire or erection. Patients must be educated to ask questions and to inform their provider of

Table 1
Cardiac disease by risk category

Low risk	Intermediate risk	High risk
Asymptomatic	Individuals with high risk	Unstable angina
<3 risk factors for CAD	categories that need further	Uncontrolled hypertension
Controlled hypertension	treatment to shift into the	Class III/IV CHF
Stable angina	low risk category	Recent MI (<2 weeks)
Successful post	≥3 risk factors for CAD	High risk arrhythmia
revascularization	Moderate/stable angina	Cardiomyopathy
Uncomplicated MI	Recent MI (>2 weeks	Severe valvular disease
Mild valvular disease	<6 weeks)	
Class I CHF		

Abbreviations: CAD, cardiovascular disease; CHF, congestive heart failure; MI, myocardial infarction.

any changes in sexual functioning between visits. Treatment may be in the form of changing medications to one that does not impair sexual functioning. The provider must ask the patient if any change in sexual function has occurred since the last visit. If the response to this question is positive, it may be a clue that the patient has stopped taking prescribed medications because of the side effects. Older adults should be questioned about the use of alcohol, as this substance alone and in combination with the prescribed medications may impact sexual functioning. Table 2 [15,16] presents the rationale and side effect of commonly prescribed medications for a patient with cardiovascular disease.

Depression

Depression is an independent risk factor for ischemic heart disease and is related to increased cardiovascular mortality. Post myocardial infarction depression is related to less compliance with medical treatment, less participation in cardiac rehabilitation, less modification of life style factors, and increased mortality. In addition, depression is associated with altering sexual desire. Cardiovascular disease has been linked with depression in numerous studies, but most specifically the literature on heart failure has reported that approximately 36% of heart failure patients become depressed. The

Table 2
Medications used by the cardiovascular patient

Drug	Rationale for use	Effect
Benzodiazepines	Sleep, antianxiety	Anticholinergic medications are associated with erectile dysfunction (ED)
Beta-blockers	Slows heart rate, decreases blood pressure	Erectile and ejaculatory problems
Calcium channel blockers	Slows heart rate, decreases blood pressure	Erectile and ejaculatory problems
Digoxin	Slow the heart rate	Decreased sexual desire
Lipid-lowering agent	Decrease cholesterol	Erectile and ejaculatory problems (participants with ED were more likely to have insulin resistance and were significantly more likely to be taking lipid-lowering medications than men without ED [15].
Thiazide diuretics	Manage hypertension	Impotence, decreased libido, failed ejaculation, and decreased vaginal lubrication [16].
Tricyclic antidepressants	Manage depression	Decreased sexual desire
Selective serotonin reuptake inhibitors	Manage depression	Decreased sexual desire, anorgasmia

numbers may actually be higher in that depression is frequently under diagnosed [17]. Depression in the cardiac population may not present as in the noncardiac patient. Typically, fatigue and insomnia are more prevalent [18]. Treatment for depression does not occur without the risk of side effects. Antidepressants, while improving the patient's depression, alleviate fatigue and insomnia, but in return decrease sexual desire. Studies are needed to identify interventions that can relieve depression and improve sexual desire among both genders.

Genital sexual dysfunction

Erectile dysfunction (ED) can occur as a risk factor, result of cardiovascular disease, or complication of prescribed medication. The causes of ED are thought to be associated with hypertension-induced injury to endothelial cells, resulting in the inability of the sinusoids of the corpus cavernosum to dilate properly. Approximately 68.3% of men with hypertension have been found to have some degree of ED. A trend was noted that those patients being treated with diuretics and beta-blockers had a higher incidence of ED, as compared with those being treated with an alpha-blocker [19]. In cardiovascular disease, a number of antihypertensives can cause erectile and ejaculatory problems. Treatment for ED is complicated as a result of many patients also using nitrates to control chest pain. Nevertheless, health care providers are often placed in a position of having sildenafil citrate (Viagra; Pfizer Inc, New York, NY) requested by the patient. Health care providers that prescribe sildenafil citrate do so with the instruction that coadministration of a nitrate along with sildenafil will result in hypotensive effects [20].

Left ventricular assist device

Circulatory assist technology facilitates the patient returning home to await a heart transplant. The left ventricular assist device (LVAD) improves the patient's condition and ultimately places the patient in position to resume a more normal life. One study reported an increase in sexual desire following implant of a LVAD [21]. While this is a small study the implications are tremendous. Specifically, patients with an LVAD need education and sexual counseling. Patients should be encouraged to explore their sexuality by slowing returning to increased sexual functioning.

Sexuality and coronary disease

Studies have shown that doctors [22] and nurses [23] do not provide the level of sexual counseling that patients need. Patients have stated that they would like the chance to discuss sexual function through a full sexual history, and that they had a high level of comfort with the topic. Historically, women receive less information about sexuality than their male counterpart who has cardiovascular disease. Evidence exists that women who live with chronic illness are concerned with sexuality [24]. There remains a lack of nurse-to-patient and doctor-to-patient discussion of sexual health. This may be a result of a lack of knowledge and skills to provide information to the patient and their partner.

Nurse's role in promoting and maintaining the patient's sexual health

Even though nurses believe that sexuality assessment should be part of their role, patients are not being assessed. In a study conducted by Magnan, Reynolds and Galvin [23], approximately 72% of the nurses believed they should discuss sexual concerns with the patient, but only 33% actually made time to address patient sexual issues. Numerous barriers exist in nurses addressing patient sexuality, such as a lack of time and heavy workload, discomfort talking about the subject, and a lack of knowledge and skills in approaching the subject.

A study conducted on 393 subjects with CVD who were surveyed regarding sexuality found that 64% of the women and 81% of the men felt that the topic of sexual functioning should be discussed. Only 18% of the women and 3% of the men felt that that they had been adequately informed about sexual functioning by their doctor [22]. Hence, nurses are often in a position to conduct an assessment of patients and they should include a full sexual history.

Approaching a patient about sexual issues must be handled with direct questioning by the health care provider, given that most people believe that sexual issues are not to be discussed. By being direct, you as the health care provider give the patient permission to openly discuss sexual concerns. Preface the discussion with the patient by stating that you are conducting a complete assessment, including sexual history, at the beginning of your examination. Use open-ended questions such as, "What problems are you having with your sexual functioning?" Be prepared for the answer to be "none." Nevertheless, make a follow-up statement that sometimes medications that have been prescribe may contribute to changes in sexual function or desire. Then ask, "Have you noticed any changes in sexual desire or function since being on your medications?" If the patient is being vague, rephrase their statement in such a way as to add specifics and seek confirmation or ask for clarification of your understanding.

Through an approach such as the PLISSIT Model [25], a nurse can uncover concerns that a patient may not necessarily identify. The PLISSIT Model (Table 3) is a guide for sexual counseling that is arranged in four levels of intervention, ranging from giving permission to discuss sexual concerns, to providing limited information, to providing specific information and referral for intensive therapy approach. With the cardiac patient, the first level of "permission" can be used to encourage discussion of sexual functioning related to cardiovascular disease and medications prescribed. At this level, the health care provider can also ask the patient about

Table 3
PLISSIT model

P = Permission to discuss sexual concern
LI = Limited Information is provided
SS = Specific Suggestions are given to enhance sexual relations
IT = Intensive Therapy is arranged

Data from Refs. [25,29,30].

relationships and the impact of their health on any sexual difficulties. Questions such as, "Do you have difficulty achieving orgasm?" or "Do you have difficulty obtaining and maintaining an erection?" should be asked by the provider [26]. At the second level, limited information can be provided to the patient and significant other on the impact of cardiovascular disease on sexual functioning. At this level, more specific questions can be presented related to loss of desire. At the third level are specific suggestions: the health care provider can provide printed material, such as the American Heart Brochures, "Sex and Heart Disease" [27] or "Sex after a Stroke" [28]. Suggestions, such as providing recommendations that reduce energy expenditure during sexual intercourse, and offering strategies to enhance intimacy through touch, hand holding, and communication of desires should be provided. Education should inform the client that sex should be avoided after meals, after excessive alcohol intake, or in extreme temperature, or following a fatiguing day. Suggestions may include treatment through sexual counseling, medications, and relationship counseling. The last level is "intensive therapy." At this level a referral should be obtained to an expert counselor, psychologist, social worker, or psychiatrist [29]. Intensive therapy should be used when an individual continues to identify sexual issues as a concern. The American Association of Sex Educators, Counselors and Therapists provide a list of resources for individuals seeking further counseling at www.aasect.org.

Couples seeking counseling because of sexual issues need to find a counselor with experience in dealing with alterations in sexual functioning caused by chronic illness [30]. Counselors need to evaluate how important sex has been in the relationship, how their sexual relationship has changed since the chronic illness, and how they are intimate with each other. The answer to these questions can help start a dialogue which can facilitate uncovering the major issues, such as fatigue, body image, gender roles, genital sexual dysfunction, severity of the disease, and medical treatment.

Summary

Even though sexual desire declines after age 75 [10], those individuals with cardiovascular disease are often required to change to adapt sexual desire to exertional limitations imposed by the disease state. Even though the American Heart Association has attempted to address sexuality through publications for the lay person, the topic is often first brought forward by the nurse during the last days of care before discharge from the hospital. Patients experiencing cardiovascular disease may have reduced sexual desire, impaired sexual arousal, erectile dysfunction, difficulty reaching orgasm, or an alteration in orgasmic intensity. These sexual issues can only be uncovered through a complete sexual history. Further research is needed to identify interventions which can benefit how both men and women experience alterations in sexual performance because of cardiovascular disease.

References

[1] Moller J, Ahlbom A, Hulting J, et al. Sexual activity as a trigger of myocardial infarction. A case-crossover analysis in the Stockholm Heart Epidemiology Program (SHEEP). Heart 2001;86:387–90.

[2] American Heart Association (2007). Statistics. Available at: http://www.americanheart.org/presenter.jhtml?identifier=4478. Accessed June 4, 2007.

[3] Carroll JL, Wople PR. Sexuality and gender in society. New York: HarperCollins; 1996.

[4] Masters WH, Johnson V. Human sexual response. Boston: Little Brown; 1966.

[5] Morgan P, Saucer C, Torg E, Editors of PREVENTION Magazine Health Books. The female body: an owner's manual. Emmaus (PA): Rodale Press; 2000.

[6] DeBusk R, Drory Y, Goldstein I, et al. Management of sexual dysfunction in patients with cardiovascular disease: recommendations of the Princeton consensus panel. Am J Cardiol 2000;86(2):175–81.

[7] Nemec ED, Mansfield L, Kennedy JW. Heart rate and blood pressure responses during sexual activity in normal males. Am Heart J 1964;92:274–7.

[8] Wagner N. Sexual activity and the cardiac patient. In: Green R, editor. Human sexuality: a health practitioner text. Baltimore (MD): The William & Wilkins Company; 1975. p. 172–9.

[9] Bohlen JG, Held JP, Sanderson O, et al. Heart rate, rate pressure product and oxygen up take in four sexual activities. Am Heart J 1984;92:274–7.

[10] American Association of Retired Persons. AARP/Modern maturity sexuality study. Washington, DC: Author; 1999.

[11] Gelfand MM. Sexuality among older women. J Womens Health Gend Based Med 2000;9(1): S15–20.

[12] Kessenich CR, Cichon MJ. Hormonal decline in elderly men and male menopause. Geriatr Nurs 2001;22:24–7.

[13] Pangman VC, Sequire M. Sexuality and the chronically ill older adult: a social justice issue. Sex Disabil 2000;18:49–59.

[14] Samelson DA, Hannon R. Sexual desires in couples living with chronic medical conditions. The Family Journal: Counseling and Therapy for Couples and Families 1999;7(1):29–38.

[15] Malmusi D, Guaraldi G, Martínez E, et al. Sexual dysfunction in HIV-infected men: prevalence and associated factors. Program and abstracts of 7th International Workshop on Adverse Drug Reactions and Lipodystrophy in HIV. 13–16 November, Dublin (Ireland): 2005 [abstract: 97].

[16] Stevenson JG, Umstead GS. Sexual dysfunction due to antihypertensive agents. Drug Intell Clin Pharm 1984;18:113–21.

[17] Faris R, Purcell H, Henein MY, et al. Clinical depression is common and significantly associated with reduced survival in patients with non-ischemic heart failure. European Journal of Heart Failure 2005;4(4):541–51.

[18] Freeland KE, Lustman PJ, Carney RM, et al. Underdiagnosis of depression in patients with coronary artery disease: the role of nonspecific symptoms. Int J Psychiatry Med 1992;22(3): 221–9.

[19] Burchardt M, Burchardt T, Baer L, et al. Hypertension is associated with severe erectile dysfunstion. J Urol 2000;164:1188–91.

[20] Kloner R. Erectile dysfunction and hypertension. Int J Impot Res 2007;19(3):296–302.

[21] Samuels LE, Holmes EC, Petrucci R. Psychological and sexual concerns of patients with implantable left ventricular assist devices: a pilot study. J Thorac Cardiovasc Surg 2004;127: 1432–5.

[22] Bedell SE, Duperval M, Goldberg R. Cardiologist's discussion about sexuality with patients with chronic coronary artery disease. Am Heart J 2002;144(2):239–42.

[23] Magnan MA, Reynolds KE, Galvin E. Barriers to addressing patient sexuality in nursing practice. Dermatol Nurs 2006;18(5):448–54.

[24] Koch T, Telford K. Constructions of sexuality for midlife women living with chronic illness. J Adv Nurs 2001;35(2):180–7.

[25] Annon JS. Behavioral treatment of sexual problems: brief therapy. Hagerstown (MD): Harper & Row; 1976.

[26] Nusbaum MRH, Hamilton CD. The proactive sexual health history. Am Fam Physician 2002; 66(9). Available at: www.aafp.org/afp/20021101/1705.html. Accessed April 7, 2007.

[27] American Heart Association. Sex and heart disease. Dallas (TX): American Heart Association; 2001.

[28] American Heart Association. Sex after stroke. Dallas (TX): American Heart Association; 2003.

[29] Annon JS. The PLISSIT model: a proposed conceptual scheme for the behavioral treatment of sexual concerns. J Sex Educ Ther 1976;2(2):1–15.

[30] Wallace M. Sexuality. Urol Nurs 2005;25(5):373–4.

NURSING
CLINICS
OF NORTH AMERICA

Nurs Clin N Am 42 (2007) 605–619

Intimacy and Multiple Sclerosis

Linda A. Moore, EdD, APRN, BC (ANP, GNP), MSCN[a,b]

[a]School of Nursing, College of Health and Human Services, University of North Carolina
at Charlotte, 9201 University City Boulevard, Charlotte, NC 28223, USA
[b]Multiple Sclerosis Center, Carolinas Medical Center, 1000 Blythe Boulevard,
Charlotte, NC 28203, USA

Multiple sclerosis (MS) is a chronic disease with progressive pathology that results in symptoms that affect, or potentially affect, all aspects of daily living and quality of life. For persons with multiple sclerosis and their partners, maintaining intimacy and sexuality is one dimension of quality of life that can be particularly challenging, and includes physical, social, and emotional issues that must be confronted. Physically, sexual function and dysfunction raise concerns throughout the disease trajectory that are common to both genders, as well as some that are gender specific. Socially, issues concerning fulfilling and maintaining family roles, parenting, and pregnancy are complex and life long consequences. Emotionally, maintaining a sense of closeness to one's significant other, in the presence of symptoms, tests a couple's ability to remain intimate. Merriam-Webster's on-line Dictionary [1] defines being intimate as: "to communicate delicately and indirectly, or a very personal or private nature." Intimacy, for persons with progressive neurologic diseases such as MS, is essential for their overall well being, but one that many often difficult to discuss with their healthcare provider, whom they perceive may not consider the intimacy problems as a priority [2].

Intimacy issues comprise those that are common across genders, as well as those that are gender specific, and are of greater or lesser importance across the lifespan and disease progression. Men are often concerned with erectile dysfunction, retrograde ejaculation, being a financial provider, and the physical demands of being a "good father." Women, on the other hand, are concerned with sensation during intercourse, menstruation, pregnancy's physical effects, menopause, and being a "good mother." Up to 50% of females and 75% of males report sexual dysfunction during the course of the disease [3]; however, it has been estimated that as many as

---

E-mail address: lmoore@uncc.edu

doi:10.1016/j.cnur.2007.07.007   *nursing.theclinics.com*

85% actually have sexual dysfunction [4]. Achieving sexual intimacy requires navigation through a complex, entangled, and dynamic set of disease processes, symptoms, and treatments that must be carefully balanced and adjusted so that intimacy, an important aspect of health, can be maximized. This article reviews the disease process, symptoms, and treatment of MS as it relates to sustaining physical, social, and emotional intimacy.

Overview of multiple sclerosis and treatment

More than 400,000 people in the United States are currently diagnosed with MS, and approximately 85% of those are in the early phase of MS, which is characterized by relapsing remitting multiple sclerosis [4]. MS is a life-long progressive process that does not decrease longevity but typically causes cognitive and physical disability, which is what leads to one of the many symptoms: sexual dysfunction. The disease pathology results in demyelination of neurons in the central nervous system, both brain and spinal cord, causing disruption in the neuronal transmission. While the cause of MS is unknown, it has been shown that there is an imbalance in the immune system between inflammatory and anti-inflammatory T-cells. Thus, activation of the immune system releases pro-inflammatory cytokines, which then target and destroy the myelin sheets that surround the nerve cells, resulting in the damage of MS. Table 1 indicates the subtypes and characteristics of the disease process [4].

Without treatment during the early stages of relapsing remitting (RR) MS, persons can expect they will move to secondary progressive (SP) MS within 15 years. In this SPMS stage, persons with MS often need the use of assistive devices for mobility. It is predicted from research data that use of pharmacologic immunomodulator therapies of interferon beta-1b (Betaseron), interferon beta-1a (Avonex and Rebif) and glatiramer acetate (Copaxone), if used in early stages of RRMS, can delay disease progression to SPMS considerably [4]. The interferons (Avonex, Rebif, and Betaseron) are injected either once a week, three times a week or every other day, depending on the particular drug. Each of the interferons decrease relapses and new brain lesion demyelination by as much as 30% through a mechanism of inhibiting inflammatory cells from entering the central nervous system (CNS). Glatiramer acetate also decreases new brain lesions, decreases relapse rates, and reduces nervous system inflammation, it is thought, by stimulating anti-inflammatory cells that enter the CNS and by restoring cytokine balance [5]. For those who have failed the previously described medications during the relapsing phase of MS, Tysabri (natalizumab) has been approved as a once a month intravenous infusion [6].

To better understand the impact of MS on physical intimacy, sexual dysfunction can be divided into three categories: primary, secondary, and tertiary. Primary sexual dysfunction results from pathologic damage in the central nervous system, especially parenchymal atrophy in the pons [7–9].

Table 1
Subtypes if multiple sclerosis

Subtypes of MS	% of total MS	Characteristics	Current disease approved treatment
Relapsing-remitting (RRMS)	85%	Relapses of neurological symptoms, followed by periods of recovery when symptoms abate with and without residual disability	Avonex IM every week Betaseron SQ every other day Copaxone SQ every day Rebif SQ 3 times a week Tysabri IV once a month
Secondary-progressive (SPMS)	(50%) of RRMS progress to SPMS	Initially RRMS course that changes over time with fewer relapses, but continued progression of the disease process; about 50% will progress to SPMS in about 10–15 years. Assistive devices, such as canes or walkers, may be required	Novantrone chemotherapy IV every 3 months
Primary-progressive (PPMS)	3%–4%	Slow and steady progression of the disease with symptoms, and no periods without symptoms with more disability. Personal care and use of wheelchairs more common	None
Progressive-relapsing	Data varies	Initially a progressive course, but then exacerbations occur. A combination of symptoms from SPMS and PPMS.	Novantrone chemotherapy

Abbreviations: IM, intramuscular; IV, intravenous; SQ, subcutaneous.
Data from Halper J, editor. Advancerd Concepts in Multiple Sclerosis Nursing Care. New York, NY, Demos Medical Publishing Inc., 2001.

Additionally, there is evidence that hormonal issues may be an important part of primary sexual dysfunction [2]. With numerous neurotransmitters that respond to both neuronal and hormonal stimuli, the exact mechanism of neurotransmission is unclear, as it relates to all aspects of pathology related to hormones in primary sexual dysfunction. The resulting pathology leads to changes in libido, decreased sensation and lubrication for women, and decreased ability for erection and ejaculation in men. Secondary sexual dysfunction arises from MS symptoms, including bladder dysfunction, fatigue, pain, cognitive dysfunction, and mobility issues. Tertiary causes are psychologic in nature [2] and are primarily related to attitudes and feelings about sexuality that are compounded by the interaction of the disease process and society's norms about sexuality [10,11].

As MS progresses, sexual functioning and intimacy become more complex for persons with MS and their partners to maintain and sustain, as does their work status, changes in parenting roles, requirements for day-to-day activities, and their physical, social, and emotional needs for intimacy.

Intimacy and symptom management

A wide range of symptoms associated with MS affect a person's ability for intimacy. Symptoms include fatigue, spasticity, tremors, cognitive ability to process information, changes in sensation (eg, numbness, pain, and decreased sensation), depression, and bladder and bowel dysfunction.

These various symptoms affecting sexual intimacy and their management are briefly discussed below, with recommendations for treatment. Initially, nurses and health care providers (HCP) should develop an organized method for evaluating sexual functioning and client concerns. One specific instrument used for assessing sexual intimacy and dysfunction in persons with MS was adapted from Szasz's Sexual Health Assessment Framework [12]. This assessment tool is useful as a starting point for discussing sexual intimacy with patients and their partners. It includes assessing sexual knowledge, sexual self-view, sexual activity, sexual response, and sexual interest and behavior [13]. The questionnaire asks whether specific symptoms occur or not and when they started. This includes areas in libido and arousal, ability at erection and orgasm, painful intercourse, and embarrassment. The questionnaire also considers medical history, as many other medical problems (eg, diabetes mellitus, hypothyroid, spinal cord injuries) contribute or are the cause of sexual dysfunction. The final section of the questionnaire asks about personal habits (eg, smoking, alcohol use, recreational drugs, and psychologic issues). From this a more comprehensive sexual assessment is made to consider MS, as well as other causes, to determine the most appropriate management plan [13].

Fatigue

A majority (75%–95%) of persons with MS describe fatigue as the number one symptom that is problematic in managing day-to-day activities, creating a cycle where fatigue, day-to-day activities, and intimacy can spiral downward. Persons with MS often report difficulty in engaging in physically intimate activities simply because of being too tired and having to struggle to stay awake. Reporting fatigue to the patient's provider is central to a complete evaluation, to determine whether fatigue stems from the MS, either as progression of the disease or as an on-going symptom, or from another coexisting condition. Treatment options should be based on determination of the underlying reason for the fatigue.

Fatigue can be described as both physical and psychologic. The physical fatigue occurs when individuals require naps during the day—either in the morning, afternoon, or both—in order to accomplish independent activities of daily living, such as shopping, house keeping, and maintaining their quality of work at the work setting. Often physical fatigue is a result of the body's response to heat in the environment. MS persons usually react very negatively to heat (eg, warm climates, rooms, and hot tubs) and should consider activities or equipment to enhance cooling activities (eg, air conditioning, cooling vests). Maintaining a cool environment assists individuals in handling some of the negative effects leading to fatigue [4]. Psychologic fatigue occurs from either depression or stress in attempting to maintain a "normal life" while managing the intermittent or constant symptoms, such as spasms, tremors, pain, bladder or bowel dysfunction, or memory and process dysfunction. Treating the symptom helps to decrease the fatigue; however, using an antidepressant that also improves energy (eg, Wellbutrin and Effexor) in the mornings can help with fatigue and depression [14].

Other physical factors leading to fatigue are related to the physical expenditure of energy. This energy expenditure most often arises from two common sources: muscle spasticity and exertion from conducting daily activities. The frequent muscle contractions seen with spasticity consume a great deal of energy, leading to fatigue. Since these contractions are not under conscious control, therapies are aimed toward minimizing the discomfort and include splinting, physical therapy, and medication [15]. These treatments are explored in more detail later in this article.

The second most common source of energy expenditure resulting in fatigue comes from exertion. Learning to plan daily activities to conserve energy is key to reducing fatigue and enhancing intimacy. Developing a schedule of activities for the day allows persons with MS to identify and prioritize activities that are essential to be completed. Persons with MS may need help in identifying alternative ways to accomplish day-to-day activities and may assist them in ensuring adequate rest, so they may have energy to engage in intimacy. For example, persons living in a two story house who find a need to go up and down stairs numerous times, may find that having a small box at both ends of the stairs, to store items that need to be placed in the direction opposite the basket, decreases multiple stair climbing and thereby conserves energy. If planning is not a skill that has been developed, making a list and scheduling activities may provide structure that can help with planning a course of action, leading to energy conservation to reduce fatigue. Learning and adhering to list-making techniques is critical to the person with MS in accomplishing tasks with the least amount of energy expenditure and enabling them to plan time for intimate activities [15].

Maintaining optimal physical function also conserves energy. Referral to physical or occupational therapy holds potential as an effective strategy for persons with MS, in learning appropriate exercises to maximize function while learning ways to conserve energy. Pacing activities and having specific rest periods supplement the skills learned in physical and occupational therapy. In order to maintain the benefit of physical and occupational therapy, the skills learned need to be continued at home. Many times this requires that family or friends help with specific exercise techniques. Additionally, learning yoga and enrolling in one of the aerobic swimming programs designed for persons with MS, are forms of exercises that have dual function in decreasing fatigue: one that enhances physical function while generating the least amount of heat because of the cooling effect of water [16].

Strategies to manage fatigue in person with MS may result in conflicting consequences. For instance, persons with MS frequently resort to drinks or medications that contain caffeine. While this does help with wakefulness, the caffeine creates additional problems that are manifested in symptoms related to bladder dysfunction. Therefore, taking caffeine as a stimulant is usually discouraged.

When energy conservation techniques (eg, planning activities, therapy, exercise) are not reducing fatigue, adding medications to the management modalities may be useful. While few medications have been approved for fatigue in MS, some insurance companies now recognize that fatigue is a major problem and have approved some of the stimulants in order to provide quality of life and help individuals maintain a normal and productive routine. A mild stimulant that many prescribe is amantadine [17]. Originally given to help prevent outbreaks of flu or reduce the symptoms of flu, this antiviral medication actually had a side effect of increased wakefulness (more commonly called insomnia). It can be given as 100 mg two times a day, with the last dose given early in the afternoon instead of at bedtime. Problems with long term use of amantadine include swelling of the feet and legs and a significant discoloration of the lower extremities, different from the rubor that persons with MS experience. In either case, the medication is discontinued, but since the discoloration (livedo reticularis) can affect body image, patients need to understand that the discoloration may take an extensive amount of time to clear [18].

Other stimulants have also been found to be effective. Interestingly, these stimulants are the same medications used for persons with attention deficit hyperactivity disorder or ADHD. Not all insurance companies approve modafinil (Provigil) at 200 mg one time a day for MS fatigue. Another set of medications come with different brand names and include the amphetamine salts (Adderall) and methylphenidate (Ritalin and Concerta). It is important to start with a low dosage and go slowly with these medications, to avoid adverse effects and to keep the dosage at the lowest level possible. While the exact mechanism of how these medications help persons with MS is unknown, it is thought that they help to conserve energy while maintaining the wake cycle. Clinical evidence shows that these medications are of major importance to persons with MS, allowing them to manage a nearly normal life. By conserving energy and staying awake, people also have more time for intimacy [19].

Depression

Depression among persons with MS affects intimacy and sexual responsiveness. In MS, depression has both physiologic and psychologic components. The interaction of these sources presents challenges to the provider in helping the person with MS manage symptoms. More than 50% of persons with MS have major depressive episodes and some of these are related to the location of lesions in the brain. Since perception of sensation is primarily a central nervous system process, lesion location can affect sensation perception. This can make sexual intercourse be perceived as painful or having little or no sensation at all [20]. The psychologic foundation for depression is multifaceted, with contributions arising from symptoms such as fatigue, realities stemming from living with a chronic illness, and struggles associated with day-to-day management. Taken together, the sources of depression can be difficult to manage. Counseling and use of medications therapy can be used in combination. Some of the selective serotonin reuptake inhibitors (SSRI) such as Prozac, as well as other antidepressants, such as Wellbutrin and Effexor, not only help with alterations in mood, but also help to enhance energy. Wellbutrin, with similar structure to amphetamine, or Effexor with norepinephrine effects, work well for energy effect and must be taken in the morning to prevent disruption of sleep [18]. For both the person with MS and his or her partner, managing depression can enhance intimacy and allow for closer relationships [20].

Numerous medications that may be required to manage other symptoms, also contribute to sexual dysfunction. It is well know that SSRIs tend to affect sexual intimacy. To counter this, changing medications to an alternative therapy may work. However, if the SSRI is really benefiting the person, consulting with the HCP for the addition of Wellbutrin may be more effective. With or without prescribed antidepressants, the question should always be asked about alternative and complimentary therapies as some of these (ie, St. John's Wort) can worsen the ability of sexual intercourse and the additive effect to other antidepressants may be detrimental [18].

Spasticity or spasms

During intimate times, it becomes distracting to both partners when muscle groups required for cuddling or sexual intercourse do not cooperate. Persons with MS commonly report that their muscles suddenly, and for no apparent, reason can spasm, and the muscle either flexes or extends. Similarly, muscle spasticity can occur where a limb refuses to relax. These involuntary reactions are neither planned nor controllable.

To minimize these annoying and interfering symptoms, physical therapy may be beneficial where learning exercises, use of splints, or leg and wrist weights may ameliorate symptoms. Additionally, medications may be prescribed by the HCP to help control muscle spasms and spasticity. Some of the medications typically used are muscle relaxers (eg, baclofen or tizanidine) and antiseizure medications (eg, gabapentin). Frequently, a combination of these medications is required to control the spasticity and spasms. Because no one medication can be predicted to work for everyone, a trial and error approach agreed on by the HCP and person with MS is used to balance control of symptoms while minimizing side effects. However, many of the medications used to control spasms and spasticity cause fatigue or muscle weakness, which may in turn compound the problem of overall fatigue, and the cycle that is a barrier to intimacy continues [21,22]. An additional treatment has been the use of botulinum toxin (Botox) for specific muscle spasticity, that usually lasts 3 to 4 months after injections [22].

When spasticity and spasm become problematic, couples can explore the pros and cons of various sexual positions that can be used during physically intimate times. Often, persons with MS report that the more traditional sexual positions may increase spasms and spasticity, so consideration for positions, such as side lying and male entrance from behind, has worked for many individuals. For women who experience severe lower extremity spasticity, mobility of legs proves to be very difficult. Improving the sexual experience may include taking the baclofen or tizanidine about 20 minutes before intercourse, and then having the male partner lie on his side, with the woman having her legs over the top of the man's legs and hips. While this seemingly awkward position decreases the close contact needed for kissing, it can provide very satisfactory intercourse. For men with lower extremity spasticity, an alternative approach is to have his partner assume the top-lying position. Sex therapy has been suggested as a method for persons with MS to determine additional methods to enhance sexual activity [23].

Pain

Persons with MS may suffer from neuropathic pain that arises from spasms, spasticity, or from the CNS electrical signals causing burning, tingling, or numbness of various parts of the body. More often these sensations are felt in the lower extremities and the perineal area. Pain in the perineal area definitely has a direct affect on sexual intimacy. It is very difficult to enjoy sexual intimacy when a previously pleasant and positive experience now causes pain. Occasionally, pain can also occurs as trigeminal neuralgia (from cranial nerve V), which makes kissing and close oral contact very painful. Currently, the best treatment for neuropathic pain has been a variety of antiseizure medications (Neurontin, Lyrica, Keppra, Depakote, Zonegran, Tegretol, Carbatrol, or Topamax) and from other medications, such as amitriptyline (Elavil). All of the medications described that help manage neuropathic pain do so through central nervous system action, the location of the major problem in MS patients with pain perception. Opioids also have a place in pain management; however, care in screening and management must be a high priority when opioids are prescribed [24].

Controlling pain requires both physical and psychologic energy to manage, which directly and indirectly impacts quality of life and the ability to maintain intimacy. Similar to the challenges associated with the pharmacologic management of fatigue, trial and error in managing neuropathic pain is needed to determine the best treatment regime that manages pain without creating another set of symptoms that can interfere with intimacy. The most common side effect from the antiseizure medications and amitriptyline is somulence, which then further creates a problem for sexual intimacy. Feeling too tired or sleepy contributes to lack of interest or ability in sexual intercourse [23]. It must be remembered that not all of these medications have Food and Drug Administration indications for neuropathic pain, and even less for the neuropathic pain of MS, and are therefore considered "off label" use and must be discussed with the patient. Other forms of pain management include using hot or cold packs for only 20 minutes, two to three times a day. Response to therapy determines which is better for each individual. At times, altering between cold and hot proves more effect than either cold or hot individually. Other therapies that have been found to be effective include acupuncture or acupressure, massage therapy, biofeedback, and limited chiropractic therapy. Most pain does not require the use of narcotics and they should be used only after other methods have been tried and failed. All aspects of neuropathic pain can contribute to a decrease in sexual intimacy, from the pain of trigeminal neuralgia to pain with intercourse. Medications and other methods have been beneficial in improving sexual relations by decreasing or eliminating the pain [11].

Bladder and bowel dysfunction

Physiologic process related to bladder and bowel dysfunction hampers intimacy and often results in unwanted disruptions during intimate situations. Urinary urgency, frequency, and bladder incontinence are problems that can be encountered. To avoid these unpleasant disruptions, simple strategies are often effective. For instance, managing intake of fluids by amount, type, and time of day can help with potential incontinence and urgency. Avoid beverages with caffeine that exacerbate urinary urgency and incontinence. In addition to avoiding caffeinated beverages, alcoholic beverages and those containing aspartame are known to irritate the bladder and increase the risk for incontinence [2]. One over-the-counter alternative therapy that has proven effective in decreasing urgency and frequency is the drug known as Prelief, which is a calcium-based product. For problems that are refractory to simpler methods, there are prescription medications (Ditropan, Detrol, Vesicare, Enablex, Sanctura, and Oxytrol patches) that help control bladder dysfunction, improving quality of life and enhancing sexual intimacy. For prescription medicine that is taken once a day, optimum results from the medication may require coordination between the times of day urinary symptoms tend to occur with the times of the peak action of the medication.

For some persons with MS, the problems associated with bladder dysfunction that can interfere with sexual intimacy are specifically related to hesitancy in starting urination and inability to completely empty the bladder. These symptoms can cause pressure from a distended bladder, creating discomfort for both men and women during sexual activity. For this, the most common treatment is with alpha-blocker medications (eg, Flomax), traditionally used for men with benign prostate hypertrophy. While this drug is considered "off-label" use for women, its action on the bladder muscle has been shown to be clinically effective for both men and women with MS. For persons with MS who utilize catherization to empty the bladder, selecting the time just before sexual intimacy provides comfort and assurance of no incontinence. Engaging in sexual intercourse with an indwelling urinary catheter is possible, but care must be taken to not dislodge the catheter. This additional concern may influence sexual satisfaction and couples may choose to experiment with sexual positions where the catheter provides less interference [25,26].

Bowel dysfunction can also be a factor in not being able to fully enjoy sexual intimacy. Constipation limits sexual satisfaction because of the general discomfort associated with an over-distended bowel. Increasing fiber in the diet, obtaining a prescription for MiraLax or a less harsh laxative can decrease the over-distended bowel. However, in order to eliminate stool it is necessary to have intact enervation of the lower thoracic cord (T6-T12). For those patients with MS in the thoracic spine, this then becomes problematic [25], and requires more aggressive management of stool elimination, which should be discussed with the HCP.

Sexual function

Regardless of gender, there are common issues that present themselves as problematic for both men and women with MS in achieving a sexually satisfying experience. Most notably, men and women experience changes in sensations that lead to sexual excitement and ability to have an orgasm. The location of brain and spinal cord lesions determines the actual physical affects on sexual dysfunction. Zorzon, Zivadinov and Boxco [27] reported the frequency of sexual dysfunction in females. Orgasmic problems occur most frequently (37%), followed by decreased vaginal lubrication (36%), and reduced libido (31%). For women on medications that affect hormones, decreased estrogen contributes to vaginal dryness and urethra irritation. Obtaining an estrogen vaginal cream from the HCP may enhance sexual intimacy. Trying over-the-counter lubricants (eg, Replens) is also a simple remedy for vaginal dryness and may be all that is necessary for some women. Education by the HCP must include information on the rationale for not using petroleum-based products; only water-based products should be used for lubrication. Few females benefit from oral medications, such as sildenafil (Viagra) [28]. Complimentary and alternative therapies, such as the compound mixture of sildenafil and L-Arginine may be beneficial in enhancing sensation [29].

Men, as well as women, with MS experience decreased sensation. For men the most common problems are with erection and maintenance through completion of orgasm. Most men have found that medications such as Viagra, Cialis, and Levitra are very beneficial. Men with MS report that if they are planning on a long weekend to spend with their partner, Cialis works best. These medications allow for the erection to occur with erotic and physical stimulation and enhance erectile function [4]. A disadvantage, in addition to the cost and the limited quantity that insurance companies will allow on prescription plans, is the potential of a significant decrease in blood pressure. Therefore, for those taking any form of nitroglycerin or alpha-blockers (eg, Flomax or Cardura), the medications listed above are not routinely recommended. There is also a delayed response in developing erections of 30 to 60 minutes after taking one of the sexual enhancing medications; therefore, persons with MS must plan ahead [18].

Not all symptoms of sexual dysfunction are attributable to MS. Many times the cause is the medication taken for the treatment of other disease processes, such as hypertension. Taking beta-blockers has been shown to decrease sexual function in both men and women. Therefore, it must be remembered to consider all medications that are necessary before assuming that MS is the cause of the problem. Additionally, changes in sexual intimacy occur because of the natural aging process, use of alcohol, smoking, lack of exercise, and illicit drug use [2]. Whatever the cause of sexual dysfunction, communication between partners is essential to manage any issues of sexual intimacy. Because one major function of intimacy is for child bearing, child rearing is an important inclusion when discussing sexual intimacy.

Child bearing and child rearing

Typically, MS causes no impairment in fertility unless the male has retrograde ejaculation [20] or either gender person is taking some forms of chemotherapy (eg, cyclophosphamide, mitoxantrone) known to alter fertility. Traditional therapeutic agents used to treat MS (Axonex, Betasereon, Rebif, and Copaxone) do not alter fertility; however, it is recommended these medications be stopped approximately 3 months before deciding on a family because of their unknown affect on fetal development. During the last trimester of pregnancy, women will notice a significant improvement in their MS symptoms. However, they are at very high risk of exacerbation within the first 3 to 8 months after delivery; therefore the HCP and the new mother should plan for immediate follow-up and potential prophylactic treatment at time of delivery or shortly thereafter. Depending on the onset of MS and the lifecycle of the family development, child rearing can be more or less physically and emotionally exhausting. Fatigue associated with the disease raises considerable issues for raising children. Likewise, as the disease progresses, the deterioration of a parent's physical and cognitive abilities can place additional stress on the family as a unit. Researchers over time have found mixed explanations as to whether stress causes exacerbations or not [30–32]. To date no clinical research has determined whether the

Table 2
Symptoms of MS and management for enhancing intimacy

Symptoms	Medical management	Patient and partner education
Fatigue	Amantadine Provigil Methylphenidate Adderall	1. Avoid hot tubs, hot showers, and activities in extreme hot temperatures 2. Maintain cool environment including cooling vests, air conditioning 3. Schedule activities to conserve energy from lists to do in priority 4. Maintain exercise program to maximize physical abilities
Depression	The following help with mood and fatigue caused by stimulating effect: Prozac or other SSRIs Wellbutrin Effexor	1. St. John's Wort for mild depression, but never in combination with prescribed antidepressants 2. Communication with partner 3. Counseling 4. Exercise releases endorphins to increase mood
Spasticity and spasms	Baclofen Tizanidine Gabapentin	1. Exercise, especially stretching 2. Taking medications for spasms about 20 min before planned intimacy 3. Alternative positions for intercourse: ie, side lying 4. Use of arm and leg weights to control spasms 5. Cuddling as an alternative to intercourse
Neuropathic Pain	Anti-seizure medications (some are off label use for neuropathic pain): Neurontin Lycrica Keppra Depakote Zonegran Tegretol Topamax Elavil	1. Communication with partner about discomforts and position changes or stimulation changes 2. Acupuncture 3. Acupressure 4. Massage therapy 5. Biofeedback 6. Decreasing fatigue and spasms can help decrease sensations of pain
Bladder dysfunction	Urgency and frequency: Ditropan Detrol Vesicare Enablex Sanctura Oxytrol patches Hesitancy or retention of urine: Flomax	1. Empty bladder before intimacy and drink glass of water after intercourse to help decrease urinary track infections 2. If using catheter, be sure to tape out of the way with intercourse

(continued on next page)

Table 2 (*continued*)

Symptoms	Medical management	Patient and partner education
Bowel dysfunction	Mild laxative	1. Have a routine for bowel elimination 2. Distended bowel can cause discomfort with sexual intercourse, as well as possible leakage
Lack of sensation for females	Vaginal lubricants Estrogen creams Compound medication of sildenafil and L-Arginine	1. Physical stimulation before intercourse, must communicate desire of stimulation and best location for stimulation to partner 2. Treating previously desired symptoms
Males and lack of sustained erection and organism	Viagra Cialis- effects last longer Levitra	Stimulation before intercourse Treating previously described symptoms Care with taking drugs and cardiac conditions requiring other drugs

results of stress are the cause of the exacerbation or whether stress leads to pseudo-exacerbation.

Facilitating symptom management to enhance intimacy

Sexual intimacy for persons with MS requires consideration of many interrelated factors. The location and number of brain and spinal lesions have a major impact on sexual intimacy and function. The medications that one takes, as well as treatment for other conditions, can also contribute to dysfunction. It is important to remember, however, that treatment for MS is the best way to help slow progression of the disease and decrease symptoms. Careful follow-up with the HCP can enhance quality of life and assist in making sexual intimacy more fulfilling. Because as many as 65% to 85% of persons with MS have sexual dysfunction, this is a major issue for health care providers to discuss with their clients. People may be reluctant to ask, so HCPs must take the first step by including sexuality in their assessment at each patient visit. Human beings enjoy being close and expressing their caring and love in various ways. For persons with MS, this may require education about causes and effects and methods to handle issues that bring alterations in sexual intimacy. The goal for persons with MS is to enhance quality in all areas of life by slowing the progression of the disease. This requires collaboration among client, family, and health care providers. Table 2 may provide a resource to symptom management to facilitate to educate MS patients and their partner in ways to enhance intimacy.

As with any physical and psychologic chronic problem, multiple sclerosis requires various combinations of therapies and treatment modalities to manage. The symptoms associated with MS are not present all of the time and do not occur to all persons with MS. Understanding one's body and needs provides the initial step toward quality intimacy.

References

[1] Available at: http:www.m-wcom/cgi-bin/dictionary. Accessed March 3, 2007.

[2] Lowden D, O'Leary M, Steverson B. Sexuality issues in patients with MS. Multiple Sclerosis Counseling Points 2005;1:1–9.

[3] Hennessey A, Robertson NP, Swingler R, et al. Urinary, fecal and sexual dysfunction in patients with multiple sclerosis. J Neurol 1999;246:1027–32.

[4] Halper J, editor. Advanced concepts in multiple sclerosis nursing care. New York: Demos Medical Publishing Inc; 2001.

[5] Wekerle H. Immunology of multiple sclerosis. In: Compston A, Ebers G, Lassmann H, et al, editors. McAlpine's multiple sclerosis. 3rd edition. New York: Harcourt Brace Co; 1998. p. 379–407.

[6] Miller DH, Soon D, Fernando KT, et al. MRI outcomes in a placebo-controlled trial of natalizumab in relapsing MS. Neurology 2007;68:1390–401.

[7] McDougall AJ, McLeod JG. Autonomic nervous system function in multiple sclerosis. J Neurol Sci 2003;215:79–85.

[8] Foley FW, Werner MA. Sexuality. In: Kalb R, editor. Multiple sclerosis: the questions you have—the answers you need. 3rd edition. New York: Demos Medical Publishing; 2004. p. 297–328.

[9] Holland N, Cavallo P. Sexuality and multiple sclerosis. NeuroRehabilitation 1993;3:48–56.

[10] LaRocca NG, Sorensen P. Cognition. In: Kalb R, editor. Multiple sclerosis: the questions you have—the answers you need. 3rd edition. New York: Demos Medical Publishing; 2004. p. 205–32.

[11] Halper J, Holland NJ, editors. Comprehensive nursing care of multiple sclerosis. 2nd edition. New York: Demos Medical Publishing; 2002.

[12] Szasz G. Sexuality in persons with severe physical disability: a guide to the physician. Can Fam Physician 1989;35:345–51.

[13] Springer RA, Clark S, Price E, et al. Psychosocial implications of multiple sclerosis. In: Halper J, editor. Advanced concepts in multiple sclerosis nursing care. New York: Demos Medical Publishing Inc; 2001. p. 213–37.

[14] Costello K, Halper J, Harris C. Nursing practice in multiple sclerosis: a core curriculum. New York: Demos Medical Publishing Inc; 2003.

[15] Clinical Practice Guidelines for Managing MS Fatigue. MS Exchange, Teaneck (NJ): International Organization of Multiple Sclerosis Nurses; August 2001. p. 3.

[16] Karpatkin HL. Multiple sclerosis and exercise: a review of the evidence. International Journal of MS Care 2005;7:36–41.

[17] Schapiro RT. Symptom management in multiple sclerosis. 2nd edition. New York: Demos Medical Publishing Inc; 1999.

[18] Lehne R. Pharmacology for nursing care. 6th edition. St. Louis (MO): Saunders; 2007.

[19] Fatigue and Multiple Sclerosis: Evidenced—Based Management Strategies for Fatigue in Multiple Sclerosis. Teaneck (NJ): International Organization of Multiple Sclerosis Nurses; PVA 1998.

[20] Kalb RC, LaRocca NG. Sexuality and family planning. In: Halper J, Holland NJ, editors. Comprehensive nursing care in multiple sclerosis. 2nd edition. New York: Demos Medical Publishing; 2002. p. 123–40.

[21] van Oosten BW, Truyen L, Barkhof F, et al. Choosing drug therapy for multiple sclerosis: an update. Drugs 1998;56:555–69.

[22] Harris CJ, Halper J. Multiple sclerosis: best practices in nursing care. 2nd edition. Teaneck (NJ): International Organization of Multiple Sclerosis Nurses; BioScience Communications; 2004.

[23] Griswold GA, Foley FW, Halper J, et al. Multiple sclerosis and sexuality: a survey of MS health professionals' comfort, training, and inquiry about sexual dysfunction. International Journal of MS Care 2003;5:37–8, 44–51.

[24] Guarino AH, Cornell M. Opioids as a treatment option for MS patients with chronic pain. International Journal of MS Care 2005;7:10–5.

[25] Chia Y, Fowler C, Kamm M, et al. Prevalence of bowel dysfunction in patients with multiple sclerosis and bladder dysfunction. J Neurol 1995;242:105–8.

[26] Morgante L, Namey M, Walker T. Bladder and bowel management. Multiple Sclerosis Counseling Points 2006;1:1–10.

[27] Zorzon M, Zivadinov R, Boxco A, et al. Sexual dysfunction in multiple sclerosis: A case-control study. Multiple Sclerosis 1999;5:418–27.

[28] Dasgupta R, Wiseman OJ, Kanabar G, et al. Efficacy of sildenafil in the treatment of female sexual dysfunction due to multiple sclerosis. Journal of Urology 2004;171(3):1189–93.

[29] Allen A. Clinical benefits of L-Arginine in achieving maximum sexual performance. Arginine Research. Available at: www.arginineresearch.com/L-Arginine.htm. Accessed June 18, 2007.

[30] Warren S, Greenhill S, Warren KG. Emotional stress and the development of multiple sclerosis: Case-control evidence of a relationship. Journal of Chronic Diseases 1982;35:821–31.

[31] Franklin GM, Nelson LM, Filley CM, et al. Cognitive loss in multiple sclerosis: Case reports and review of the literature. Archives of Neurology 1989;46:162–7.

[32] Fisher JS, Foley FW, Aikens JE, et al. What do we really know about cognitive dysfunction, affective disorders, and stress in multiple sclerosis: a practitioner's guide. Journal of Neurologic Rehabilitation 1994;8(3):151–64.

ELSEVIER
SAUNDERS

NURSING
CLINICS
OF NORTH AMERICA

Nurs Clin N Am 42 (2007) 621–630

Arthritis and Sexuality

Ann Mabe Newman, RN, DSN

School of Nursing, College of Health and Human Services, University of North Carolina at Charlotte, 9201 University City Boulevard, Charlotte, NC 28223, USA

What is arthritis?

More than 120 kinds of arthritis exist. In addition to the more common types of musculoskeletal disorders such as osteoarthritis (OA), rheumatoid arthritis (RA), and osteoporosis, arthritis also includes fibromyalgia, Paget's disease, gout, polymyalgia rheumatica, septic arthritis, bursitis, rotator cuff tears, drug-induced systemic lupus erythematosis, and Sjogren's syndrome [1]. Although all forms of arthritis may interfere with the activities of daily living, including intimacy, the focus of this article is on OA and RA because they are more common. Because RA, in particular, can be severe, it can result in difficulties of employment and put a stress on family relationships [2].

RA is characterized as a chronic, progressive, inflammatory condition that primarily affects the joints, with damage to ligaments, tendons, cartilage, and joint capsule [3]. By contrast, OA results in cartilage degeneration, and bone regeneration (growth) may result in bone spurs. RA symptoms are symmetric (wrists, knees, knuckles), whereas OA symptoms usually result in localized pain and stiffness (bony knobs on end joints of fingers, and usually not much swelling) [2]. Treatment for RA consists of reducing inflammation, a balanced exercise program, joint protection, weight control, relaxation, heat, medication, or surgery. Treatment for OA includes maintaining activity level, exercise, joint protection, weight control, relaxation, heat, medication, or sometimes surgery [2].

Taboos surrounding the impact of arthritis on people's sex lives

An article in the current *Arthritis Today*, the leading lay publication sponsored by the Arthritis Foundation, leads with this screaming byline in caps, "YOUR SEX LIFE - OR THE LACK THEREOF - MAY NOT BE A TOPIC THAT GETS MUCH AIRTIME DURING AN

E-mail address: amnewman@uncc.edu

APPOINTMENT WITH YOUR RHEUMATOLOGIST." But maybe it should [4]. Among health care providers, the assumption is often made that people who have arthritis do not want to talk about their sex lives. However, nothing could be further from the truth. In a recent study by Ryan and Wylie [3], they assert that ".....patients would welcome the opportunity to discuss their sexual needs with a health professional" [3]. The researchers sought to identify the current perceived practice, skills, and knowledge of rheumatology nurses in addressing the sexuality of patients with RA. They found that 69% of the nurses felt that sexuality should be included in the nursing assessment. Nurses reported that contraceptive advice for patients treated with cytotoxic drugs was discussed in depth, but the patient's sexual relationship was not discussed at all. Most of the nurses (83%) had never received any education in this area but would undergo training if they had the opportunity. Because patients who have arthritis want someone to talk to about their sexual issues and most nurses do not feel qualified to discuss sexual issues, sexuality and arthritis remain very much a taboo subject.

Sexual functioning of people who have arthritis

Literature on the sexual functioning of people who have arthritis can be characterized as old and scant. Indeed, a literature search of the topic was dismal, and yet, sex is a normal part of the everyday lives of most people. Panush and colleagues [4] note that their awareness of the lack of literature on sexual dysfunction in people who have arthritis came from a *Penthouse* publication. Panush and colleagues also note that, of the few research articles available on the topic, "only 10 studies adequately assessed sexual function in rheumatic disease patients. Even these few studies were limited by not having definitions, indices, or validated methods for evaluating sexual difficulties for people with rheumatic disease." Little has changed since this article was published in 2000.

Nevertheless, the effects of the disease itself can affect the person's sex life because of pain, fatigue, and depression. These symptoms can be compounded by the effects of the medications used to treat the chronic condition [4]. Sexual functioning may also be affected by the loss of self-esteem, which may accompany living with rheumatic diseases [5–9]. The attitudes of others, particularly one's partner, may also contribute to sexual dysfunction.

Osteoarthritis

OA of the hip and knee are two of the most common causes of pain and disability in adults [10]. Some researchers estimate that between 70% and 85% of people more than 55 years of age have OA [10]. Although OA is more prevalent than RA, recent research on sexual dysfunction has been directed more toward the latter. With the aging of the baby boomers, this situation is likely to change.

Two thirds of people with hip OA experience sexual problems [11], making it fertile ground for nursing research and evidence-based care. OA causes pain, tenderness, and limitation of movement, and therefore, it can have a negative effect on a person's ability to enjoy sex. Twenty-five percent of people with OA report they have some marital difficulty with regard to their sex lives, related to the effect of pain and stiffness, as opposed to the effects of libido [4].

Rheumatoid arthritis

Inflammation and fatigue, two of the symptoms associated with RA, can have a major effect on a person's sex life. The statistics on the devastating effects are overwhelming: 50% of people with RA experience loss of interest in sex; 60% are unsatisfied with their quality of life related to sexuality; 85% of women and 69% of men with RA report that joint swelling with associated symptoms is a major factor in their decision about whether or not to initiate sex [4].

In a study comparing men and women with RA to controls regarding sexual motivation, activity, satisfaction, and specific problems, the researchers also sought to determine the correlation of the physical aspects of the disease with sexual functioning [12]. The researchers found that male patients experienced less sexual desire, and female patients fantasized and masturbated less than the controls. However, no differences in satisfaction were found, and male and female patients did not report more sexual problems than controls. Age, sexual motivations, and activities correlated in the women, and physical health and sexual problems correlated among the men. Fifty-one percent of the women and 41% of the men reported having trouble with several joints during sexual activity. The researchers conclude that patients with RA are less active sexually than the controls and men and women have problems with their joints during sexual activity. The researchers further conclude, however, that sexual satisfaction did not differ between those with RA and the control group [12]. The physiologic changes caused by RA are probably independent of the psychologic changes. The investigators also argue that "sexual satisfaction also depends on personal and social factors. In men, physical health and disease activity are more related with sexual problems than in women" [12].

Another recent study attempted to determine the clinical and psychologic factors significantly contributing to sexual disability and dissatisfaction in female patients with RA [13]. Sixty-two percent reported difficulties with sexual performance. Of that number, 17% were totally unable to engage in sexual intercourse because of their arthritis. Sexual desire or sexual satisfaction were reported as "diminished" by 46% of the subjects and as "completely lost" by 46% of the RA patients. Psychodemographic variables did not significantly correlate with sexual disability. However, sexual disability correlated with parameters of disease activity; disability as measured by the widely used Health Assessment Questionnaire (HAQ); hip, but not knee, joint disease; seropositivity; and diminished desire [13]. The "HAQ-disability and hip joint disease were the only independent and significant determinants of sexual disability in the regression model after controlling for the effects of age and disease duration" [13]. Sixty-four percent of the variance of sexual disability was explained by these variables together. The researchers note that, by contrast, pain, age, and depression were the significant determinants in the regression model for sexual dissatisfaction, and all together contributed 36% of its variance [13]. The researchers conclude that sexual disability and diminished sexual desire and satisfaction are experienced by more than 60% of female patients with RA. Overall hip disability and hip involvement related more to difficulties in sexual performance, whereas perceived pain, age, and depression influence diminished desire and satisfaction more [13].

Medications and their influence on sexual dysfunction in arthritis

A number of medications are used to treat arthritis that may interfere with sexual functioning [4]. The high doses of glucocorticoids, which are commonly used to treat many forms of arthritis, may have side effects that affect the sexual functioning of people who have arthritis. The characteristic "buffalo hump," the moon face, and thin extremities may affect personal self-esteem. Decreased libido, depression, mania, and psychosis may also result from the use of glucocorticoids. Immunosuppressants may also have an effect on sexuality, in the form of oral and genital ulcers, skin rashes, anemia, and hair loss. Hair loss in particular may contribute to an increasing loss of self-esteem caused by living with the chronic symptoms of arthritis. Additionally, cyclophosphamide, one of the immunosuppressives, can result in amenorrhea and infertility [4].

Patient and partner issues related to sexuality

Couples living with pain and fatigue when one partner suffers from arthritis face challenges in keeping their relationship alive and well, especially intimacy, so cherished by all couples [2]. Although sexuality is expressed in very individual ways by people who have arthritis, some generalizations have been observed [4]. Society's expected gender roles for men include strength and gainful employment. Arthritis may alter this role, leaving the man vulnerable to depression and altered self-esteem. Likewise, women are expected to be wife, mother, and nurturer, and, in today's economy, income provider. When the woman who has arthritis is not able to meet society's expectations, or even her own expectations, her self-esteem tends to decrease. And, as noted earlier, sexual activity tends to decrease. Pain, fear of pain, and fatigue tend to decrease libido. When partners fear they are causing pain, they tend to not initiate intercourse or to try to get it over with as quickly as possible to avoid further injury, which further exacerbates the problem.

In a study to determine predictors of marital and sexual satisfaction in patients with RA and their spouses, 59 patients and their spouses completed questionnaires independently of each other [14]. Demographic variables, disease status, psychologic distress, and social support were correlated with marital and sexual satisfaction. The researchers conclude that "psychological distress and social support are more important than objectively assessed disease status in determining marital and sexual satisfaction in patients with RA" [14]. Clearly, more research on the topic needs to be done.

Communication

In real estate, it is said that the three most important things in buying a house are location, location, location. The three most important things for a successful sexual relationship for people who have arthritis are communication, communication, communication [2]. In the widely used *The Arthritis Helpbook*, the writers suggest that when one has a chronic condition such as arthritis, good communication becomes a necessity [2]. They admonish, "Your health care team, in particular, *must* understand you. It is in your best interest as a self-manager to learn the skills necessary to make your communications as effective as possible" [2]. People who have arthritis frequently are frustrated because they may not have visible signs of their illness to signal their pain and fatigue. "You don't understand" is the frequent culmination of a conversation between a person who has arthritis and his/her partner in regard to sexuality. Therefore, it is paramount to ensure that the person who has arthritis has the skills to take control of his/her illness before the subject of using specific techniques for a more satisfying sex life is initiated. The author has devoted the better part of the last 25 years of her career to helping people who have arthritis learn effective communication skills as a part of self-management, to feel empowered in dealing with their illness [15].

Effective communication begins with listening, and learning to express one's own feelings [16]. Learning to use "I" messages is a fundamental concept in feeling heard and understood. Any good text on communication skills or assertiveness training will give the practitioner help in teaching these techniques. However, every nurse who is attempting to teach these techniques to clients should engage in a period of self-reflection to ensure that he/she has mastered the techniques himself or herself. Teaching assertiveness and self-management requires the nurse to have high self-efficacy for teaching these skills if he/she is to be successful in teaching them to persons who have arthritis. As noted in the study cited earlier, most nurses do not feel they possess these skills. Teaching persons who have arthritis how to communicate with the health care team is a precursor to learning effective communication skills; likewise, the health care team must possess these skills before they can teach them. Only as this interactive process is mastered by client and nurse can conversations regarding sexuality begin.

Lorig, who has devoted her career to helping people feel more in control of their arthritis, offers excellent suggestions for approaching the topic of sexuality in *The Arthritis Helpbook* [2]. Her comments are addressed to clients in an easy-to-read, supportive manner. Nurses who wish to help clients who have arthritis and their partners enjoy a more satisfying sex life would do well to read and emulate her approach of placing sexuality in the context of intimacy, as she describes techniques for overcoming fear, for sensuality with touch and fantasy, for overcoming pain during sex, and for sexual positions for people who have arthritis.

Specific strategies

Sex is supposed to be pleasurable, but if fear of being in pain or causing pain is on the mind of either partner, it can be frustrating. For human beings, the sharing of physical and emotional sensuality can be as important as the act of sexual intercourse. Making love versus "having sex" can actually improve sex if couples are willing to explore new and different ways of physical and emotional stimulation [2]. Again, open communication is the key to strengthening any relationship. A helpful phrase the author teaches couples who are trying to learn to communicate more openly is "I feel _____ when you _____, and what I need from you is _____." As couples explore open communication with regard to intimacy, the blanks might be filled in with "I feel *sad* when you *are ready for sex and I'm not,* and what I need from you is *a lot more foreplay.*" This communication obviously sounds artificial to most people, but doing it in a playful manner can set the stage for more serious discussions on how to make sex more comfortable [16].

For most people who have arthritis, it is the act of sexual intercourse that is the most difficult to sustain [2]. Therefore, spending time arousing your partner can make lovemaking last longer and still be satisfying. We tend to forget that climax can occur without intercourse and, in fact, for most women it is more pleasurable. Sharing the pleasure of lovemaking may be more important than climax for some people. "No matter how or if climax is reached, pain due to activity or position is minimized if we concentrate on foreplay and sensuality rather than intercourse itself" [2].

Dealing with fear

Part of the fear associated with pain comes from the fact that, once it has been experienced, it may return, and even be worse, the next time. People who have arthritis have difficulty managing their daily lives with the pain they experience and when pain is associated with sex, guilt adds to the burden. The partner of the person who has arthritis may feel even more guilty and selfish that he or she may be responsible for increasing the pain during sex. This guilt may turn into resentment. Again, communicate, communicate, communicate. It is the unspoken words that get people in trouble. Without open communication, it is impossible for couples to experiment with new positions. The health professional should teach couples to start with simple phrases such as "I like it when we are able to talk like this; then I don't feel so scared that I'm going to hurt you," or "I like it when we can talk like this; then I don't feel so scared that my pain is going to keep us from enjoying sex."

When, and only when, partners are comfortable talking about sex, can they begin to talk about what kinds of stimulation they prefer and what positions are most comfortable [2]. This kind of conversation does not happen easily for most couples. "I can't say THAT, he'll think I'm a slut," one woman confessed to the author. Actually, she reported back to the author that her husband found it to be a real turn-on when she was able to say, "I like it when you touch me there," or "Moving the pillow under my hips makes your penis go in easier." This same women was so embarrassed by her joint deformities that giving her permission to make love in the dark was all it took to decrease her fear of rejection.

Touch

The skin is the largest sensual organ of our bodies because it is rich with sensory nerves. Erotic feelings can be aroused by the right touch on almost any area of the skin [2]. People who have arthritis can find a comfortable position and enjoy the sexual stimulation that comes with touch. Flavored oils, lotions, feathers, fur gloves, any of these things can be used to increase arousal. In addition to the use of the hands, many people are aroused when touched by the lips, tongue, or sex toys. "Vibrators can be very helpful in creating arousal and even climax with minimal physical demands" [2].

Creating fantasies

At some time or the other, most people engage in fantasies and it is considered to be perfectly normal. However, for some couples, this issue becomes sensitive if the idea has not been explored before lovemaking occurs. Engaging in fantasy does not mean comparing your partner to someone more attractive. It does not mean the partner would rather be with a glamorous media or sports idol. It can be enjoyable to explore mutual fantasies out of the bedroom and then try them out during lovemaking, even if it is as simple as saying something you know your partner likes to hear during sex [2].

Dealing with pain and fatigue

Sometimes no amount of foreplay, touch, or fantasy will help the person who has arthritis find a comfortable position for sex. The accompanying fatigue experienced by people who have arthritis compounds the problem. This situation has the possibility of recreating the scenario described earlier (pain causing the partner who has arthritis to feel resentful that he/she did not climax, guilt and frustration about being an inadequate partner, lowered self-esteem), and so the cycle continues until the person begins to avoid sex, which can exacerbate the problems for both partners.

One helpful thing nurses can do is suggest to the person who has arthritis to time his/her medication so it will reach its maximum potential when sex is planned. Being cognizant of the type of medication the client is taking is also important. Narcotics and muscle relaxants can cause dulling of the sensory nerves, which may decrease the enjoyment of sex. Other types of pain medications can be used if this becomes a problem. Teaching couples to plan for sex can help with the problem of fatigue. Sometimes, a short nap, a warm bath, or planning for sex in the mornings can help the client conserve energy for lovemaking. Couples may complain this planning takes away from the spontaneity of sex, but sometimes, planning for an activity can make it more exciting [2].

In the author's practice with people who have arthritis, she has found that teaching relaxation techniques is one of the best ways to break the cycle of pain and fatigue. Again, self-reflection and perceived competence on the part of the nurse in teaching these techniques require that the nurse herself must learn the techniques. Mastering the techniques is not easy, but to have credibility with clients, one must be willing to "walk the walk." The relaxation response techniques created by the work of Benson and Klipper [17] in the 1970s continue to be helpful to clients (and the author, too). The four basic elements to the relaxation response are

- A quiet environment
- An object or word to dwell on
- A passive attitude
- A comfortable position

Based on some of the same principles as meditation, the steps used to elicit the relaxation response include

1. Sit quietly in a comfortable position with your eyes closed. Try to tune out internal and external distractions.
2. Breathe in through your nose and, as you breathe out through your mouth, try to empty your mind of distracting thoughts by saying the word one to yourself.
3. Continue for 10 to 20 minutes. When you finish, sit quietly for a few minutes with your eyes closed before standing up.

The client should not worry about doing it "right," but should just continue to maintain a passive attitude, and when distracting thoughts occur, dismiss them and return to repeating the word one. The relaxation response techniques should be practiced once or twice a day. It may take several weeks of concentrated practice before the client feels he/she is making progress, but it will come.

Finding a comfortable position

Before the person who has arthritis and her/his partner are too aroused to want to change positions during sex, they need to practice some positions beforehand. Finding positions that are comfortable for both partners can be considered part of foreplay. Experimentation is the key to finding the right position because all people are different [2].

Many books and pamphlets are available for helping clients find the least painful positions for sex. The absolute best source of information for clients/patients is "A Guide to Intimacy with Arthritis," an 8-page, illustrated reprint from *Arthritis Today*, the publication from the Arthritis Foundation. It offers helpful and forthright information, including position modifications for more comfortable sex, and can be purchased from your local Arthritis Foundation [18].

In addition to the publication, a Web site with the same title, *Guide to Intimacy with Arthritis*, uses a panel of qualified experts (a rheumatologist, a person with arthritis, a psychologist, and a registered nurse) to answer questions related to sex, posed by Web site readers who have arthritis. The answers are directed toward the topics

- It's too painful
- Decrease in desire
- Sex and flares
- New joints
- Getting creative
- Moisture problems
- Body image
- Scared of infidelity
- Starting over
- Get what you need
- Sex as a painkiller
- Talking about it
- Where to find help

The Web site can be found at: http://www.arthritis.org/resources/relatioships/intimacy/experts/asp.

Summary

People who have arthritis can have satisfying sex. Clients may need to be taught to be creative and be willing to experiment. Good communication and planning are necessary for people who have arthritis and their partners to have a satisfying sexual relationship.

General recommendations to clients for having a more satisfying sex life are

- Communicate needs/wants to partner.
- Practice relaxation, fantasizing, guided imagery.
- Take pain medication to peak when sexuality activity will occur.
- Take a warm shower, or use heat before sex, to increase muscle relaxation.
- Practice positions before sexual activity.
- Stop and change positions or rest during sexual activity.
- Explore alternative ways to express intimacy.
- Use alternative ways of bringing partner to orgasm (masturbation or oral-genital sex).

References

[1] Luggen AS, Meiner SE. Introduction. In: Luggen AS, Meiner SE, editors. Care of arthritis in the older adult. New York: Springer; 2002. p. 1–8.

[2] Lorig K, Fries JF. Arthritis: what it is. In: The arthritis helpbook. 6th edition. Cambridge (MA): Da Capo Press; 2006. p. 3–14; 286–90.

[3] Rayan S, Wylie E. An exploratory survey of the practice of rheumatology nurses addressing the sexuality of patients with rheumatoid arthritis. Musculoskeletal Care 2005;3(1):44–53.

[4] Panush RS, Mihaillescu GD, Wallace DH. Sex and arthritis. Bull Rheum Dis 2000;49(2): 1–4.

[5] Yoshimura S, Uchida S. Sexual problems of women with rheumatoid arthritis. Arch Phys Med Rehabil 1981;62:122–3.

[6] Elst P, Sybesma T, Van Der Stadt RJ. Sexual problems in rheumatoid arthritis and ankylosing spondylitis. Arthritis Rheum 1984;27:217–20.

[7] Baum J. A review of the psychological aspects of rheumatic disease. Semin Arthritis Rheum 1882;11:352–61.

[8] Cohn M. Sexuality and the arthritic patient—how well are we doing? J Rheumatol 1987;14: 403–5.

[9] Hamilton A. Sexual problems in arthritis and allied conditions. Int Rehabil Med 1980;3: 38–42.

[10] Birchfield P. Osteoarthritis. In: Luggen AS, Meiner SE, editors. Care of arthritis in the older adult. New York: Springer; 2002. p. 11–27.

[11] Morely JE, Tariq SH. Sexuality and disease. Clin Geriatr Med 2003;19:563–73.

[12] van Berso WT, van de Weil HB, Taal E, et al. Sexual functioning of people with rheumatoid arthritis: a multicenter study. Clin Rheumatol 2007;26(1):30–8.

[13] Abdel-Nasser AM, Ali EI. Determinants of sexual disability and dissatisfaction in female patients with rheumatoid arthritis. Clin Rheumatol 2006;25(6):822–30.

[14] van Lankveld W, Ruiterkamp G, Naring G, et al. Marital and sexual satisfaction in patients with RA and their spouses. Scand J Rheumatol 2004;33(6):405–8.

[15] Newman AM, et al. Effects of self-help program on women with arthritis. In: Funk S, Tournquist E, Champagne M, editors. Key aspects of chronic pain: hospital and home. New York: Springer; 1993. p. 122–7.

[16] Newman AM. Self-concept. In: Boggs K, Arnold E, editors. Communication in nursing. Philadelphia: Saunders; 2006. p. 72–111.

[17] Benson H, Klipper MZ. The relaxation response. New York: Quill; 2002.

[18] Belmont M, Dodge, C, Ranier, J. et al. Guide to intimacy with arthritis. Arthritis Foundation. Available at: http://www.arthritis.org/resources/relatioships/intimacy/experts/asp. Accessed May 1, 2007.

ELSEVIER
SAUNDERS

Nurs Clin N Am 42 (2007) 631–638

NURSING
CLINICS
OF NORTH AMERICA

Sexuality in Chronic Lung Disease

Teresa Tarnowski Goodell,
PhD, RN, CNS, CCRN, APRN, BC

Oregon Health & Science University School of Nursing, 3455 SW US Veterans
Hospital Road SN6S, Portland, OR 97239, USA

The desire for sexuality and intimacy is a fundamental human trait that continues following the diagnosis of a chronic lung disease. There is much that health care providers can do to assist the person who has chronic lung disease in meeting needs for sexuality and intimacy. This article discusses some of the physiologic alterations that influence the expression of sexuality and intimacy as well as the psychoemotional factors that health care providers can assess and modify to promote optimal sexual health in people who have chronic lung disease.

Although chronic obstructive pulmonary disease (COPD) and lung cancer (LC) are not the only adult chronic lung diseases, they are the two most prevalent function-limiting lung diseases [1,2]. Asthma, for example, is fairly common, (more so in adult females than males) affecting over 10 million American adults [3]; but most cases of asthma are mild enough to represent little or no detriment to physical functioning. In contrast, COPD and LC are progressive and associated with declining function. These diseases share several characteristics, such as symptoms (progressive breathlessness, fatigue, anorexia, malnutrition) and etiology (smoking, toxic exposure) [4] that impact sexuality. This article is therefore devoted primarily to COPD and LC, although the recommendations for promoting healthy sexuality and intimacy may apply to adults who have any function-limiting respiratory disease.

Chronic obstructive pulmonary disease: pathophsyiology and sexuality

COPD is widely considered a smoker's disease because approximately 85% of individuals diagnosed with COPD are current or former smokers [1]. An estimated 16 million American adults have symptomatic COPD

E-mail address: goodellt@ohsu.edu

doi:10.1016/j.cnur.2007.08.003   *nursing.theclinics.com*

and many more have subclinical, undiagnosed COPD [1]. Chronic obstructive pulmonary disease is the fourth leading cause of chronic morbidity and mortality in the United States [5]. In coming years, the global burden of COPD is expected to rise due to continued exposure to risk factors (tobacco and environmental irritants) and the aging population [5].

The pathophysiologic characteristics of COPD are linked to its symptoms: airway inflammation causes mucus accumulation, expectoration, and cough; bronchoconstriction causes wheezing and diminished air movement; and air trapping due to emphysema causes shunting, limiting the amount of lung surface taking part in gas exchange and promoting hypoxemia and hypercarbia. All of these pathophysiologic characteristics contribute to shortness of breath and decreased physical endurance.

Although hypoxemia and hypercarbia are features of severe COPD, it is important to appreciate that the sensation of shortness of breath (or breathlessness) is not closely linked to measurable alterations in blood gases or pulmonary function tests [6–10]. Breathlessness is a multidimensional, multicausal subjective sensation occurring in association with changes in tissue oxygenation, chest wall compliance, muscle strength, and psychoemotional responses. Among the physiologic mechanisms contributing to breathlessness are an altered sense of respiratory effort, stimulation of lung chemo- and baroreceptors, changes in skeletal muscle physiology, and central nervous system–ventilatory dissociation (misperception of pulmonary signals by the central nervous system) [11–16].

The sensation of breathlessness is not purely physiologic; it is also linked to subjective meaning, coping, and emotions [10,15,17–21], and thus purely biomedical approaches to treating breathlessness have been criticized as incomplete [19]. Breathlessness has been called the most difficult symptom to manage in lung disease and a neglected symptom [15,20].

Chronic obstructive pulmonary disease and sexual performance issues

Impotence may influence satisfaction with sexuality and intimacy in some people who have COPD and their partners. The severity of impotence, or erectile dysfunction (ED), in men who have COPD exceeded that of age-matched controls [22], occurring to a moderate to severe degree in 57% of participants who have COPD versus 20% of age-matched controls in one study. Overall, in this study, 87% of study participants who had COPD had some degree of ED. Explanations for this finding include processes mediated by proinflammatory agents such as tumor necrosis factor alpha, a marker of global inflammatory status in COPD, which was found in substantially higher concentrations in those who had worse ED. Other studies have demonstrated the prevalence of sexuality-related problems in COPD [23,24], but most have concerned only males who had COPD. Virtually no evidence exists on intimacy and sexuality issues in women who have COPD and their partners.

Lung cancer

Approximately 170,000 Americans are diagnosed each year with lung cancer, and nearly that number die of it [2]. The high death-to-incidence ratio of lung cancer is related to difficulties associated with diagnosing the disease: most LC is diagnosed late in its progression, leaving fewer treatment options and a shorter lifespan after diagnosis in comparison to other common cancers. Lung cancer is the leading cause of cancer deaths worldwide and kills more Americans yearly than colon, breast, and prostate cancer combined [2]. Unlike COPD, LC occurs almost exclusively in older people; the great majority of individuals who have LC are over age 65 [25].

Lung cancer: pathophsyiology and sexuality

Reduced physical functioning and high physical symptom burden are well documented in LC. Fatigue, depression, shortness of breath, cough, and pain are common symptoms in lung cancer [26–28]. These symptoms influence expressions of sexuality and intimacy in various ways. Fatigue decreases the ability to engage in physical activity of any kind. Diminished physical endurance and muscle strength contribute to easy fatigability and may deter all attempts at physical sexual acts that the couple enjoyed in the past [29]. Breathlessness is a frightening experience and strongly associated with anxiety [29,30]. Fear of acute shortness of breath alone may discourage couples from engaging in sexual intercourse. Cough may be viewed as interrupting, unappealing to the partner, and as an impediment to the spontaneity of sexual expression that many couples value. Pain may be exacerbated by physical sexual expression and may be interpreted as evidence of tissue damage that should be avoided. The effects of symptoms extend to the partner of the person who has lung cancer, who may fear exacerbating symptoms, and inadvertently causing harm or discomfort through sexual activity.

Chronic obstructive pulmonary disease and lung cancer: medications and sexuality

Many medications can cause sexual dysfunction. Perhaps the most commonly implicated are vasoactive medications, such as beta-blockers, that cause ED. However, many other classes of medications can cause altered physical sexual responses and impaired libido in men and women, and many of these are in common use by people who have lung disease. Among medications often in use by individuals who have lung cancer, regardless of the cancer treatment regimen, are opioid analgesics and selective serotonin reuptake inhibitors to treat depression. Other medications have been suggested as antidotes to the sexual side effects of antidepressants [31] and may be of use if nonpharmacologic methods of meeting sexual and intimacy needs are insufficient. A complete list of medications that cause ED, compiled by the National Library of Medicine, is available at: http://www.nlm.nih.gov/medlineplus/ency/article/004024.htm. The proliferation of phosphodiesterase inhibitors, such as sildenafil (Viagra, Pfizer, New York, New York), vardenafil (Levitra, Bayer Pharmaceuticals, West Haven, Connecticut), and tadalafil (Cialis, Lilly ICOS, Indianapolis, Indiana), in recent years has offered a solution to one of the problems with sexuality and intimacy that accompany lung disease.

Unfortunately, sexual performance issues among women garner considerably less attention than those of men, and there are fewer remedies for altered physical responses to sexual arousal in women. Vaginal lubricants may be helpful to postmenopausal women, but they address only one aspect of the many changes in physical arousal that occur after menopause. Sildenafil has been tested in women and found ineffective [32], although similar biochemical pathways function in men and women to achieve physical sexual arousal. One explanation for this apparent contradiction is that subjective satisfaction with intimate and sexual function is not closely related to objective measures of physical sexual function in women, whose arousal is highly dependent upon psychoemotional factors [33–35]. This observation helps explain differences in sexual satisfaction among men who have COPD and their female partners, whose lack of satisfaction with the sexual aspects of their relationships has been attributed to declining quality of communication between the partners [24].

Women who have undergone chemotherapy for LC may experience premature menopause [36]. Alkylating agents such as cyclophosphamide, ifosfamide, cisplatin, carboplatin, and fluorouracil are associated with menopausal symptoms. These drugs have been used to treat LC for many years. Education of women, particularly younger women who have LC, about menopausal side effects, loss of fertility, and premature menopause is a crucial nursing responsibility. Men who will receive chemotherapy for LC should be similarly informed that alkylating agents also cause testicular changes. In either case, patient and partner should ideally be educated about foreseeable alterations in sexual performance and altered communication patterns within their intimate relationship.

People who have COPD and LC often have some degree of reactive airway disease, or asthma. For this condition, inhaled corticosteroids (such as beclamethasone, fluticasone and triamcinolone), anticholinergic bronchodilators (ipratropium, tiotropium), and long-acting (salmeterol) and short-acting (albuterol) sympathomimetic bronchodilators are prescribed. Proper regular use of long-acting inhaled medications helps maintain function and control the symptoms of disease. The use of a short-acting bronchodilator before physical activity improves physical performance and comfort during activity. Use of a short-acting bronchodilator before sexual intercourse should be promoted in individuals who have activity-induced bronchoconstriction.

Chronic obstructive pulmonary disease and lung cancer: specific suggestions for clinicians and patients

The threat to life and functional decline that accompany COPD and LC put enormous pressures on couples. Some respond to the stress of a serious lung disease by an increased desire for affection, intimacy, and physical expressions of sexuality. Others may suffer loss of sexual desire, emotional alienation, and diminished ability to physically perform [37]. The first step, therefore, is assessment of the individual's and couple's responses to diagnosis and treatment.

Most health care providers are aware that there are a multitude of normal differences in sexual response and desire between women and men and among individuals. These include the types of stimuli and length of time required to produce physical arousal and the frequency of sexual desire and sexual fantasies [33]. Differences in individual preferences for intimate expression are also prevalent. The diversity in human responses to sexuality and intimacy mandate that health care providers assess thoroughly and non-judgmentally for sexuality and intimacy problems in individuals who have physical illnesses. Unfortunately, many health care providers are inexperienced or uncomfortable with assessment of sexuality and intimacy.

Treatment of sexuality and intimacy issues in lung disease depends upon the primary cause of the problem. Medication side effects may be allayed by altering the drug regimen or prescribing other drugs to counteract negative effects. Unmanaged shortness of breath may be similarly decreased by altering the medication regimen and educating clients about the proper use of medications. Technique is particularly problematic with inhaled medications, which have a high rate of misuse [38–42].

Pulmonary rehabilitation programs, which typically feature exercise, respiratory muscle training, and education components, have repeatedly been shown beneficial in improving physical function in COPD [43–46]. In COPD, it is known that skeletal muscle changes associated with deconditioning, cytokine release, and malnutrition contribute to physical limitations and can be reversed with pulmonary rehabilitation [47,48]. Although these effects have rarely been studied in LC, it is likely that rehabilitation would enhance physical function in this group as well, and wider inclusion of people who have LC in pulmonary rehabilitation programs has been recommended [49].

The interference of fatigue and shortness of breath during sexual activity may be minimized by exploring alternative methods of expression with an intimate couple. Side- and bottom-lying positions may be more comfortable, for example, for the affected partner. More comfort for the affected partner may enhance the unaffected partner's enjoyment of the sexual experience

and diminish fears of exacerbating symptoms. These benefits may be sufficient to encourage the couple to try positions that one or both partners
had formerly considered unappealing.

Summary

Like COPD, lung cancer is strongly associated with smoking. However,
the relationship between smoking and lung cancer may not be as clear-cut
as commonly believed. Lung cancer advocacy organizations, in particular,
point out that only approximately 20% of smokers are ever diagnosed
with lung cancer, and over 50% of people who have LC are nonsmokers
when diagnosed [50]. Comparable statistics have been reported for COPD
[51] Underlying these statements is concern for the perceived stigma against
people who have smoking-induced illness, compared with illnesses that are
not as strongly linked to lifestyle factors [52]. This stigma has been the subject of little research, but it is potentially damaging to the psychologic well
being of people affected by the disease. Individuals who have lung cancer
experience more intense psychosocial effects than people who have other
types of cancer. This probably relates to the burden of physical symptoms
like fatigue, pain, and breathlessness; advanced stage of the illness at the
time of diagnosis; and the poor prognosis associated with LC, in addition
to perceived social stigma.

Multiple factors converge to cause sexuality and intimacy problems in
individuals who have chronic lung disease. It is imperative that clinicians
include in their discussions with patients the ways they can maintain their
sexual lives in the face of chronic lung diseases such as COPD and LC. Providing patients and their partners with information on ways to enhance their
overall physical functioning as well as discussing the many pharmacologic
and nonpharmacologic methods available to maintain healthy sexual lives
is critical to having a quality life. It is apparent that more research is needed
so that we can help people with chronic lung disease and their partners
continue to have quality sexual relationships.

References

[1] Petty TL. Chronic obstructive pulmonary disease. In: Hanley ME, Welsh CH, editors.
    Current diagnosis & treatment in pulmonary medicine. McGraw-Hill; 2003. Access-
    Medicine.com.
[2] American Lung Association. Trends in lung cancer morbidity and mortality. 2006. Available
    at: http://www.lungusa.org/site/pp.asp?c=dvLUK9O0E&b=33347. Accessed April 15, 2007.
[3] Centers for Disease Control and Prevention. Self-reported asthma prevalence among adults -
    United States, 2000. MMWR Morb Mortal Wkly Rep 2001;50(32):682–6. Available at:
    http://www.cdc.gov/mmwR/preview/mmwrhtml/mm5032a3.htm. Accessed March 26, 2007.
[4] Jantarakupt P, Porock D. Dyspnea management in lung cancer: applying the evidence from
    chronic obstructive pulmonary disease. Oncol Nurs Forum 2005;32:785–97.

[5] Fabbri L, Barnes P, Buist A, et-al. Global strategy for the diagnosis, management, and prevention of chronic obstructive pulmonary disease: executive summary. 2006. Available at: http://www.goldcopd.com/Guidelineitem.asp?l1=2&l2=1&intId=996. Accessed April 16, 2007.

[6] Heyse-Moore L, Beynon T, Ross V. Does spirometry predict dyspnoea in advanced cancer? Palliat Med 2000;14:189–95.

[7] American Thoracic Society. Dyspnea mechanisms, assessment, and management: a consensus statement. American Thoracic Society. Am J Respir Crit Care Med 1999;159:321–40.

[8] Lareau SC, Meek PM, Press D, et al. Dyspnea in patients with chronic obstructive pulmonary disease: does dyspnea worsen longitudinally in the presence of declining lung function? Heart Lung 1999;28:65–73.

[9] Dudgeon DJ, Kristjanson L, Sloan JA, et al. Dyspnea in cancer patients: prevalence and associated factors. J Pain Symptom Manage 2001;21:95–102.

[10] Dudgeon DJ, Lertzman M, Askew GR. Physiological changes and clinical correlations of dyspnea in cancer outpatients. J Pain Symptom Manage 2001;21:373–9.

[11] Manning HL, Mahler DA. Pathophysiology of dyspnea. Monaldi Arch Chest Dis 2001;56: 325–30.

[12] Demediuk BH, Manning H, Lilly J, et al. Dissociation between dyspnea and respiratory effort. Am Rev Respir Dis 1992;146:1222–5.

[13] Beniaminovitz A, Lang CC, LaManca J, et al. Selective low-level leg muscle training alleviates dyspnea in patients with heart failure. J Am Coll Cardiol 2002;40:1602–8.

[14] Gandevia SC, Butler JE, Hodges PW, et al. Balancing acts: respiratory sensations, motor control and human posture. Clin Exp Pharmacol Physiol 2002;29:118–21.

[15] Anonymous. Dyspnea in cancer patients needs more attention. J Support Oncol 2006;4: 63–4.

[16] Mador MJ, Bozkanat E. Skeletal muscle dysfunction in chronic obstructive pulmonary disease. Respir Res 2001;2:216–24.

[17] Tarzian AJ. Caring for dying patients who have air hunger. J Nurs Scholarsh 2000;32: 137–43.

[18] von Leupoldt A, Mertz C, Kegat S, et al. The impact of emotions on the sensory and affective dimension of perceived dyspnea. Psychophysiology 2006;(43):382–6.

[19] Krishnasamy M, Corner J, Bredin M, et al. Cancer nursing practice development: understanding breathlessness. J Clin Nurs 2001;10:103–8.

[20] Booth S, Silvester S, Todd C. Breathlessness in cancer and chronic obstructive pulmonary disease: using a qualitative approach to describe the experience of patients and carers. Palliat Support Care 2003;1:337–44.

[21] Carrieri-Kohlman V, Gormley JM, Eiser S, et al. Dyspnea and the affective response during exercise training in obstructive pulmonary disease. Nurs Res 2001;50:136–46.

[22] Karadag F, Ozcan H, Karul AB, et al. Correlates of erectile dysfunction in moderate-to-severe chronic obstructive pulmonary disease patients. Respirology 2007;12:248–53.

[23] Kim HFS, Kunik ME, Molinari VA, et al. Functional impairment in COPD patients: the impact of anxiety and depression. Psychosomatics 2000;41:465–71.

[24] Ibanez M, Aguilar JJ, Maderal MA, et al. Sexuality in chronic respiratory failure: coincidences and divergences between patient and primary caregiver. Respir Med 2001;95:975–9.

[25] American Cancer Society. Detailed guide: lung cancer - non-small cell. Available at: http://www.cancer.org/docroot/CRI/content/CRI_2_4_1x_What_Are_the_Key_Statistics_About_Lung_Cancer_15.asp?sitearea=. Accessed April 26, 2007.

[26] Fox SW, Lyon DE. Symptom clusters and quality of life in survivors of lung cancer. Oncol Nurs Forum 2006;33(5):931–7.

[27] Gift AG, Jablonski A, Stommel M, et al. Symptom clusters in elderly patients with lung cancer. Oncol Nurs Forum Online 2004;31:202–12.

[28] Gift AG, Stommel M, Jablonski A, et al. A cluster of symptoms over time in patients with lung cancer. Nurs Res 2003;52:393–400.

[29] Barnett M. Chronic obstructive pulmonary disease: a phenomenological study of patients' experiences. J Clin Nurs 2005;14:805–12.

[30] Bailey PH. The dyspnea-anxiety-dyspnea cycle—COPD patients' stories of breathlessness: "It's scary when you can't breathe." Qual Health Res 2004;14:760–78.

[31] Rosenblate R, Zajecka J. 2000. Treatment resistant depression: a guide for effective psychopharmacologists. Medscape Psychiatry & Mental Health. Available at: http://www.medscape.com/viewprogram/149. Accessed January 10, 2007.

[32] Basson R, McInnes R, Smith MD, et al. Efficacy and safety of sildenafil citrate in women with sexual dysfunction associated with female sexual arousal disorder. J Womens Health Gend Based Med 2002;11(4):367–77.

[33] Basson R. Clinical practice. Sexual desire and arousal disorders in women. N Engl J Med 2006;354:1497–506.

[34] Basson R. The complexities of women's sexuality and the menopause transition. Menopause 2006;13:853–5.

[35] Basson R. Female sexual response: the role of drugs in the management of sexual dysfunction. Obstet Gynecol 2001;98:350–3.

[36] Knobf MT. Reproductive and hormonal sequelae of chemotherapy in women. Cancer Nurs 2006;29:60–5.

[37] Lamb MA. Sexuality. In: Ferrell BR, Coyle N, editors. Textbook of palliative nursing. New York: Oxford University Press; 2001. p. 309–15.

[38] van Schayck CP, BijlHofland ID, Folgering H, et al. Influence of two different inhalation devices on therapy compliance in asthmatic patients. Scand J Prim Health Care 2002;20:126–8.

[39] Schiller KW. Validation of a metered-dose inhaler adherence scale with an electronic medication monitor and inhaled corticosteroid adherence and concomitant bronchodilator use in adults. Dissertation Abstracts International: Section B: The Sciences and Engineering. 2001;62-2B:1060.

[40] Erickson SR, Horton A, Kirking DM. Assessing metered-dose inhaler technique: comparison of observation vs. patient self-report. J Asthma 1998;35:575–83.

[41] van der Palen J, Klein JJ, Kerkhoff AHM, et al. Evaluation of the long-term effectiveness of three instruction modes for inhaling medicines. Patient Educ Couns 1997;32:S87–95.

[42] Allen SC, Ragab S. Ability to learn inhaler technique in relation to cognitive scores and tests of praxis in old age. Postgrad Med J 2002;78:37–9.

[43] Casaburi R. Combination therapy for exercise intolerance in COPD. Thorax 2006;61:551–2.

[44] Lacasse Y, Brosseau L, Milne S, et al. Pulmonary rehabilitation for chronic obstructive pulmonary disease. Cochrane Database of Systematic Reviews 2006;4:CD003793.

[45] Sanchez Riera H, Montemayor Rubio T, Ortega Ruiz F, et al. Inspiratory muscle training in patients with COPD: effect on dyspnea, exercise performance, and quality of life. Chest 2001; 120:748–56.

[46] Reishtein JL. Review: rehabilitation improves exercise capacity and alleviates shortness of breath in chronic obstructive pulmonary disease. Evid Based Nurs 2004;7:22.

[47] Sue DY. Peripheral muscle dysfunction in patients with COPD: comparing apples to apples? Chest 2003;124:1–4.

[48] Antonucci R, Berton E, Huertas A, et al. Exercise physiology in COPD. Monaldi Arch Chest Dis 2003;59:134–9.

[49] ATS/ERS Pulmonary Rehabilitation Writing Committee. American Thoracic Society/European Respiratory Society statement on pulmonary rehabilitation. Am J Respir Crit Care Med 2006;173:1390–413.

[50] Lung Cancer Alliance. Lung cancer facts. 2007. Available at: http://www.lungcanceralliance.org/facing/facts.html. Accessed April 26, 2007.

[51] Silva GE, Sherrill DL, Guerra S, et al. Asthma as a risk factor for COPD in a longitudinal study. Chest 2004;126:59–65.

[52] Chapple A, Ziebland S, McPherson A. Stigma, shame, and blame experienced by patients with lung cancer: qualitative study. BMJ 2004;328:1470–3.

ELSEVIER
SAUNDERS

Nurs Clin N Am 42 (2007) 639–653

NURSING
CLINICS
OF NORTH AMERICA

HIV, AIDS, and Sexuality

Mario R. Ortiz, RN, PhD, APRN, BC

Department of Nursing, Purdue University North Central,
1401 South U.S. Highway 421, Westville, IN 46391, USA

Sexuality is a part of being human and living a full life. The well-being of many individuals centers on affectionate, loving relationships that contribute to health and quality of life. Individuals who are living with a chronic illness, such as HIV/AIDS, live rich, full lives that health care professionals can support through holistic assessment and interventions. So important is the issue of sexuality that in 2001, US Surgeon General David Satcher listed "promoting sexual health and responsible sexual behavior" as one of the ten leading health indicators for the nation. Satcher initiated a national dialog on issues of sexuality, sexual health, and responsible sexual behavior. He called for the development of strategies that focus on increasing awareness, implementing and strengthening interventions, and expanding research related to sexual health matters [1].

For persons living with HIV/AIDS, sexuality is important in promoting sexual health, responsibility, and happiness. The purpose of this article is to outline information about HIV and AIDS and provide nurses with information on how to provide high-quality care for these patients related to sexuality and intimacy. This care is provided through a discussion of relationships, sexuality and sexual health, gender perceptions about sexuality, sexual needs and difficulties, and nursing assessment and intervention strategies (Box 1).

Relationships, sexuality, and sexual health

A diagnosis of HIV infection is no longer an imminent death sentence. Although there is no medical cure, HIV is currently managed as a chronic disease [2]. At the end of 2005, the Centers for Disease Control and Prevention estimated that 1 million people in the United States were living with HIV or AIDS [3]. Nurses are likely to provide care to persons living with

E-mail address: mortiz@pnc.edu

Box 1. Sexual health care in persons who have HIV

1. Assess concerns about the sexual relationship
A. Do a brief sexual assessment
  1. Concerns about sexual activity by patient and partner
  2. Current sexual activity
  3. Importance of sex in relationship
  4. Medications and health problems
B. Discuss information about sexual activity with HIV/AIDS
C. Encourage open and honest communication between the patient and partner about sexuality
D. Suggest that the couple take daily walks to improve functional capacity and promote intimacy
E. Remind the couple that the demand of sexual activity is similar to other daily activities
F. Remember that sexual activity is individually defined (eg, hugging, kissing, fondling, masturbation, sexual intercourse)

2. Discuss activity guidelines
A. Remind the couple that more general activities, such as kissing, hugging, and fondling, are safer sex activities
B. Sexual intercourse may be practice with condoms and barriers using water-based lubricants and following safe-sex guidelines
C. Encourage the couple to use foreplay before sexual activity to focus on intimacy and not just on performance

3. Address environmental issues that should be considered before sexual activity
A. Encourage a comfortable, familiar setting to minimize any stress in resuming sexual activity
B. Remind the patient that he or she should be well rested at the time of sexual activity (eg, early morning, after a nap)
C. Encourage the patient to use a comfortable position for sexual activity
D. Discourage eating or drinking 1 hour before sexual activity
E. Avoid unfamiliar surrounding or partners to minimize stress and anxiety

4. Discuss warning signs of fatigue and distress
A. Encourage the patient to report any warning signs that are experienced with sexual activity (eg, pain, shortness of breath, dizziness, insomnia, extreme fatigue the day after sexual activity)

B. Advise the patient to use medications for sexual dysfunction according to provider prescription

C. Advise the patient to notify the primary provider of any side effects that persist or cause discomfort

5. *Discuss medication effects on sexual function, individualizing it to the patient's medication plan*

A. Discuss the patient's medications and their side effects; encourage the patient to report any sexual problems promptly to the primary provider

B. Consult a current drug therapy handbook or pharmacology book for each specific medication

C. Other considerations

1. Take a sexual history before starting any new medication that might affect sexual function

2. Encourage the patient not to stop taking medications if they have a side effect. The patient should consult the primary provider. Substitution of the medication may be possible or the dosage adjusted

6. *Review guidelines for anal sex and elicit drugs*

A. Teach the patient that anal sex may lead to decreased cardiac performance and chest pain through vagal stimulation and to notify the primary provider if chest discomfort occurs

B. Avoid drugs such as stimulants, cocaine (chest pain, myocardial infarction), or marijuana (increased heart rate and myocardial oxygen consumption) because sexual dysfunction also may occur with these substances

---

HIV/AIDS; it is important that they understand the importance of sexuality to patients for whom they provide care. Sexuality pertains to all things that relate specifically to being a woman or a man. It is subject to life dynamic change as a function of total personality. It includes body image, self-esteem, and how we would like others to see us. It involves more than sexual desires, activity, and orientation. It encompasses touching, intimacy, and the physical closeness of others and can be an expression of warmth and caring, relationships, and gender roles [4].

The need for other people, love, intimacy, and the rewards of relationships and friendships is deeply personal. For some people living with HIV, the mutual love of a partner may be the most important need in their whole of life [5]. For others, friendship may be what is most valued or simply the opportunity to share personal experiences with others facing the same problems [6]. Isolation and loneliness are common experiences among people living with HIV. Relationship breakdown, bereavement, and displacement from family and friends are three of many possible causes [5]. HIV can be a particularly heavy burden for relationships and friendships to bear, and many do not survive the disclosure of HIV status [4–6]. Even when responses are supportive, the impact of HIV on personal identity, priorities, and goals inevitably has consequences for relationships of all kinds. People who choose to keep their HIV status secret may find that doing so inhibits the closeness and familiarity of their relationships [7].

Illness, treatment side effects, depression, and low self-image also can make it difficult for people who have HIV to sustain established relationships and social lifestyles [8,9]. Within sexual relationships, the infectivity and vulnerability of the individual who has HIV can radically change attitudes and behavior. The high rate of sexual dysfunction among people who have HIV also can damage relationships [10]. In all intimate relationships, whether discordant (with one person being HIV positive and the other being HIV negative) or concordant (with both persons being HIV positive), support must be given as well as received, which can be particularly challenging for people who have HIV if they are feeling vulnerable [11]. This vulnerability can be countered by having a sense of well-being reinforced by intimate relationships.

The need for sexual well-being encompasses broader needs for sexual health, sexual confidence, and sexual fulfillment [12]. For many people who have HIV, sexual well-being may be as simple as finding a sexual partner or a partner who will be with them after disclosure of HIV status. The experience and apprehension of rejection are common because they undermine self-confidence and increase anxiety about the difficulties of forming sexual relationships [13]. Beyond anxiety about other people's responses, people who have HIV also may worry about their own personal infectivity and the risk of onward transmission of HIV [13]. Personal exposure to other infections or reinfection also structures thoughts about risk during sex and individual strategies used in lowering risk. These many interrelated worries may manifest as a loss of interest in sex, a loss of enjoyment when actually having sex, or actual sexual dysfunction [14]. The physical and psychological impacts of illness and treatment side effects also can have a profound impact on sexual confidence and enthusiasm for sex, especially if they lead to changes in personal appearance [15,16]. They are also heavily implicated in the high rates of sexual dysfunction among people who have HIV [5,10,17].

The World Health Organization [18,19] also reinforced the need for sexual well-being when stressing the importance of personal rights in terms of sexuality and humanness. The organization asserted that sexual rights embrace human rights that are already recognized in national laws, international human rights documents, and other consensus statements. They include the right of all persons—free of coercion, discrimination, and violence—to

1. receive the highest attainable standard of sexual health, including access to sexual and reproductive health care services
2. seek, receive, and impart information related to sexuality
3. receive sexuality education
4. garner respect for bodily integrity
5. choose their partner
6. decide to be sexually active or not
7. have consensual sexual relations
8. enter consensual marriage
9. decide whether—and when—to have children
10. pursue a satisfying, safe and pleasurable sexual life [18]

The responsible exercise of human rights requires that all persons respect the rights of others [4]. It is important that persons who are living with HIV/ AIDS live in situations and are taken care of in ways in which the freedom to express themselves as unique, loving individuals is guaranteed and supported.

Gender perceptions on sexuality

Women

For many women, HIV creates new ways in which they live and experience sexuality. "Yet, women do not stop having sexual feelings because of a positive diagnosis. Many HIV positive women continue to have sexual relationships and desires; others choose abstinence because they find it empowering" [20]. As women with HIV live longer, healthier lives, it is essential to understand their patterns of sexual behavior, which place women, their sexual partners, and offspring at risk for sexually transmitted diseases. It is also important to focus on measures that enhance sexual health within the context of life with HIV infection. This knowledge could lead to prevention measures and interventions that enhance sexuality and sexual health among HIV-infected women [20].

In research about the influence of HIV on sexual activity and functioning in women, it was found that (1) most women continue to be sexually active after testing HIV positive, (2) sexual functioning does not change as a result of HIV disease progression, and (3) few women report that HIV itself caused worsening of their sexual functioning [21]. Higher levels of sexual functioning also were found in women with better mental health, more positive meaning attributed to a life with HIV infection, better quality of life, fewer HIV-related symptoms, and no history of use of injection drugs. Although most women continue to be sexually active after a positive HIV diagnosis, decreased sexual functioning is common and more prevalent than among HIV-positive men [22,23]. The women in this study viewed HIV as sexually inhibiting. Women discussed accounts of diminished spontaneity, foreclosed (provisional) sexual freedom, foreclosed power, foreclosed flirtation, inciting violence, (un)natural sex, responsibility imperatives, muted/mutated sexuality, and diminished intimacy [22]. These themes were reflected in these women's accounts, wherein a focus on protecting others frequently impeded their own sexual fulfillment and emotional relationships.

Men

Highly active antiretroviral viral therapy (HAART) has enabled HIV-infected men who have sex with men (MSM) to live longer. However, HAART's success means that there are more MSM living with HIV who can potentially transmit the virus to their sex partners [24]. This fact emphasizes the importance of focusing sexual health and prevention efforts on persons who are living with HIV. Although many MSM reduce risk behaviors after learning that they have HIV, most remain sexually active [24]. Most HIV-infected MSM believe that they have a personal responsibility to protect others from HIV, but some engage in risky sexual behaviors that may result in others contracting HIV [25,26]. More interventions for persons living with HIV must be implemented and researched.

Social and economic factors, including racism, homophobia, poverty, and lack of access to health care, are barriers to receiving HIV prevention services, particularly for MSM of minority races or ethnicities [27,28]. African American and Hispanic men are more likely than white men to be given a diagnosis of HIV infection in the late stages of infection, often when they already have AIDS, which suggests that they are not accessing testing or health care services through which HIV infection could be diagnosed at an earlier stage. The stigma associated with homosexuality may inhibit some men from identifying themselves as gay or bisexual, although they have sex with other men. An example of this is the "down low" phenomenon in the African American community, in which men who have sex with men and with women do not identify themselves as gay or bisexual [27]. Identifying oneself as heterosexual and having sex with men is not unique to African American men, however. These men may miss prevention and health messages directed to openly gay men, especially because African American and Hispanic MSM are less likely than white MSM to live in gay-identified neighborhoods [27]. Prevention programs directed to gay-identified neighborhoods may not reach these MSM.

For Hispanic MSM, unique cultural factors may discourage openness about homosexuality: *machismo*, the high value placed on masculinity; *simpatia*, the importance of smooth, nonconfrontational relationships; and *familismo*, the importance of a close relationship with one's family [28,29].

Preparing health care professionals to address patient sexual needs

To understand the sexual effects of HIV/AIDS on the way persons live, it is important to have a working knowledge of the pathogenesis of HIV. The HIV viruses belong to the Lentivirus subfamily of the RNA retroviruses. Like most retroviruses, the HIV genome consists of three structural genes: *gag, pol,* and *env* [30]. The *gag* gene codes for viral capsid proteins, *env* for the viral envelope proteins, and *pol* for the proteins responsible for viral replication, including the RNA-dependent DNA polymerase known as reverse transcriptase [30].

Usually, spread of the virus occurs after a break in the integument or mucous membranes. HIV infection occurs when the envelope subunit gp120 binds the human CD4 T-cell receptor found primarily on lymphocytes and monocyte-derived macrophages [30]. Binding also requires the presence on the host cell of the chemokine receptor CCR5 or CXCR4 [30]. The viral envelope then fuses with the host cell, which allows discharge of the viral core into the host cell. Viral DNA is synthesized by reverse transcriptase and integrated into the host genome by the protein integrase [31]. Once the viral gene products are transcribed and assembled, the HIV protease mediates packaging of new virions for release into serum to spread the virus [30].

Over time, infected persons have a progressive loss of CD4+ lymphocytes, although in the early stages of infection, this is not associated with increased immunosuppression. The rate of CD4 cell loss varies and depends on viral and host factors. Typically, infected persons lose 40 to 80 CD4 cells/mm^3 per year [30]. A subset of individuals advance rapidly, and 5% of infected persons, known as long-term nonprogressors, have little or no progression of clinical disease or decline in CD4 counts over 10 years, even without antiretroviral therapy [30].

Transmission of the virus occurs through exposure to contaminated body fluids, including blood, semen, and vaginal fluid [31,32]. The most prevalent modes of transmission are sexual contact (male-male or heterosexual sex), parenteral exposure to blood and blood products, and vertical transmission during pregnancy. The size of risk depends on the exposure. For example, the risk of HIV transmission from a known HIV-positive source from receptive anal intercourse is 0.1% to 0.3%, whereas receptive vaginal intercourse carries a risk per episode of 0.08% to 0.2%. A percutaneous exposure, such as a needle-stick injury or injecting-drug use, results in transmission 0.4% or 0.67% of the time, respectively [32]. The threat of vertical transmission from mother to fetus without any protective therapy is approximately 25% [33,34]. The effectiveness of transmission increases with greater degrees of viremia in the source patient and the presence of concurrent sexually transmitted diseases [32].

Assessment of sexuality and sexual health

To offer holistic care to persons who are living with HIV/AIDS, nurses should encourage people to talk about their sexuality and sexual problems [4]. As part of holistic care, nurses should assess sexual needs, particularly in patients who have HIV/AIDS. The health assessment should include questions about sexuality that explore the person's sexuality and sexual problems in the same way that other physical, psychological, spiritual, and social issues are assessed.

The nurse should be comfortable in asking questions such as

1. How has being positive affected your sexual life?
2. How has treatment affected your sexual life?
3. How has being positive interfered with your relationship?
4. How does your partner feel about your sickness?
5. How is your sexual performance during this time of illness? [4]

These are only starting points to a dialog about sexuality and sexual issues with the person. Once there is a certain level of trust between nurse and patient and the nurse continually shows that he or she is comfortable and ready to talk about the topic, the conversation can move into more specific aspects of intimacy [35–37]. Initiating the exchange assists patients in articulating concerns and feelings about sexuality, which has the potential to be therapeutic [4].

Sexual education and information on HIV

To maintain self-esteem and a healthy body image, patients who have HIV/AIDS need not only sexual activity but also touching, intimacy, and the physical closeness of others [7,38]. It is critical that persons who have HIV/AIDS and their partner receive timely and appropriate information that allows them to continue to fulfill their roles within families, achieve effective communication with their partners, maintain privacy, and enables them to make their own decisions [28,29]. People who have HIV/AIDS can have various sexual problems, including those that involve body image and self-perception, loss of libido, inability to negotiate condom use and safer sex, and sexual dysfunction [8,15,21,38–41]. Sexual feelings and expression may be inhibited by problems such as difficulty negotiating condom use, fear of reinfection or infecting a partner if that person is HIV negative, and either fear of or great desire for pregnancy [40–43].

Body image and problems of self-perception

Body image is a person's view of himself or herself. It is a personal image of one's body as seen through one's own eyes and perspective. Body image is formed by a person's experience of living with his or her body. Although everyone has an image of his or her body, each person's self-image is unique. How a person views and feels about his or her body enhances sexual well-being and promotes sexual activities. If people have negative beliefs about their bodies, as is the case for many people living with HIV/AIDS, it can interfere with their sexuality and sexual health [4,16,39,40].

Of concern, persons who have lipodystrophy may be more likely to believe that their HIV status is noticeable by the body alterations brought on by antiretroviral medications compared with persons without lipodystrophy [44]. In the post-HAART era, HIV infection and treatment with antiretroviral therapy are associated with different but significant bodily changes. In particular, the HIV lipodystrophy syndrome is a recognized complication of effective antiretroviral therapy that is characterized by often striking changes in various body fat stores, both central and peripheral. Body changes associated with the lipodystrophy syndrome include increased visceral adiposity, hypertrophy of the posterior cervical fat pad ("buffalo hump"), and subcutaneous fat atrophy at the extremities and on the face [44].

Despite notable evidence that body image can be an important factor in psychosocial well-being, medical treatment adherence, and sexual health, patients' body image concerns are not usually explicitly addressed by clinicians, even in cases of noticeable disfigurement, such as HIV lipodystrophy [45]. Such an oversight may reflect nurses' discomfort with or lack of skill at addressing such issues. The necessity for nurses to address this important issue is underlined by the damaging impact of lipodystrophy on adherence with antiretroviral therapy [44–46]. Body image screening procedures may provide a standardized method to better understand the full spectrum of body image concerns that patients experience and result in better communication between persons who have HIV/AIDS and the health care team.

Communication between a nurse and patient is crucial, especially when a person's body image and self-perception are negative and not self-appraising. These feelings may bring about feelings of worthlessness, which may make it difficult to be aroused sexually. A person's sexual partner may think that he or she is not interested in him or her sexually or is cheating if there is no interest in sex [4]. The situation may worsen if the person who has HIV/AIDS has not shared what is causing the problem. For these reasons, nurses should help patients share their experiences with their partners. This communication can be a problem, however, if the healthy partner blames the person who has HIV/AIDS for bringing the disease into the family, particularly in a discordant couple [11,28,29,47–49]. Nurses must be aware of various mental health and support group resources so that counseling and support may be offered to couples as they learn ways to communicate with each other and negotiate their relationship.

Loss of libido

Low testosterone levels noted in men with HIV infection, particularly those who have AIDS, can exacerbate existing problems with sexual functioning, mood, and energy. Some drugs used to treat HIV-related complications, notably megestrol and ketaconazole, may be a cause of lower serum testosterone levels. These low testosterone levels may contribute to decreased sexual interest and arousal [50,51]. HIV-infected women also develop a loss of libido that damages their personal relationships and negatively affects their sexual quality of life [52]. In many patients who have HIV or AIDS, sexual desire decreases because of fatigue, generalized wasting, muscle aches, pains, paresthesias, and depression. Body image concerns worsen with symptomatic disease [52].

Research has documented that protease inhibitors, such as amprenavir (Agenerase), fosamprenavir (Lexiva), indinavir (Crixivan), lopinavir/ritonavir (Kaletra), ritonavir (Norvir), saquinavir (Fortovase), and nelfinavir (Viracept), have an adverse effect on desire and arousal [53,54]. Transmission of HIV with viral loads of less than 1500 copies/mL is reportedly rare, however [52]. It is important that HIV-discordant couples practice safe sex. Nurses should examine a couple's understanding of safe-sex practices and highlight the value of using condoms, dental dams, and water-based lubricants.

Negotiating condom use

The use of condoms, especially with couples in committed relationships, is strongly associated with sex that may be occurring outside of the primary relationship [4,41–43,46]. The use of condoms fluctuates according to serostatus, age, type of relationship, and whether there are or will be children in the primary couple's life. Introducing the use of condoms into any relationship is complicated, so open, truthful communication and expression of feelings with a person's partner are vital [4,41,46,47,55]. Nurses may assist persons in discussing condom use by teaching them that a way to begin a conversation with one's partner is by introducing a safer sex conversation during a low-key moment: while on a walk, during dinner, over the phone. It is also important that a person start the conversation slowly by maybe mentioning a news story about condoms or a magazine article on sexually transmitted diseases. For persons involved in a steady relationship, he or she may say that a desire to use condoms is based on one's growing awareness of safer sex and living healthy with HIV, not a lack of trust in the relationship.

These conversations about condom use may be followed by many moments of great emotional difference, however, in which professional assistance may be needed. These emotional periods are usually related to notions of distrust between partners, especially because many persons believe that condoms are used in casual and commercial sex rather than in committed, loving relationships [4,41,46,47,55].

Safer sex

Living with HIV/AIDS has an impact on sexual relationships because safer sex techniques musr be practiced to ensure that each partner remains free of infections, sexually transmitted diseases, and possible reinfection for persons who are HIV positive [12,56]. Safer sex is the term used to describe sexual activities that minimize the risk of spreading sexually transmitted diseases. It is important that the nurse communicate that just because one partner is infected, HIV infection does not necessarily have to have a negative impact on sexual and emotional intimacy. It is important to emphasize that communicating about each person's feelings and fears is important

[35]. The nurse should point out that sensuality should take prevalence over sexuality and discuss the difference with the couple.

The nurse may lead a discussion about experimenting with safer sex activities, such as mutual masturbating, hugging and kissing, playing with sex toys, massage, and the sharing of fantasies. These activities also enhance the level of physical and emotional intimacy. Introducing latex barriers (ie, condoms, gloves and dental dams) into sex play is the easiest and most effective way to minimize the risk of transmitting bodily fluids [20]. The nurse may have to explain that a dental dam is a little square of latex that was originally designed for use by a dentist. Currently, dental dams are also widely used as a protective barrier in cunnilingus (mouth/tongue contact with female genitals) and analingus (mouth/tongue contact with the anus). Dams can be obtained from the local sex store, the dentist, or some sexologists. It is important to remind persons that they must always use a water-based lubricant when using latex. Oils and oil-based lubricants destroy rubber and render latex barriers useless.

Sexual dysfunction in patients who have HIV

Painful intercourse

There are various infections for which persons who have HIV/AIDS are at risk. The signs and symptoms of these various infections often result in pain either during or after sexual intercourse, which affects sexual functioning and intimacy. Most commonly, women are susceptible to human papillomavirus, which is a sexually transmitted viral infection that causes the abnormal growth of tissue in the form of warts or dysplasia (ie, change in the size, shape, or appearance of cells). Human papillomavirus can affect the cervix, vagina, vulva, urethra, and anus [34]. Pelvic inflammatory disease, a general term that refers to infection of a woman's internal reproductive organs (ie, fallopian tubes, ovaries, and uterus) and is often caused by untreated sexually transmitted infections, particularly chlamydia and gonorrhea, can lead to serious consequences, including infertility, ectopic pregnancy, abscess, and chronic pelvic pain. These symptoms can vary from none to severe. If symptoms are present, they can include lower abdominal pain, fever, unusual vaginal discharge, burning during urination, painful intercourse, and irregular menstrual bleeding [34].

Many women who have HIV/AIDS experience episodes of trichomonas (trich, which is a sexually transmitted infection caused by the protozoon *Trichomonas vaginalis*). Although many women experience mild to no symptoms, if symptoms are present, they can include a frothy, yellow-green vaginal discharge with a strong odor, pain during intercourse and when urinating, irritation, and itching around the vagina [34]. Finally, women who are living with HIV/AIDS are at risk for vaginal candidiasis (yeast infection, vaginitis, candida), which is a fungal infection of the vulva and vagina. Recurrent infections are the most common initial symptoms of HIV infection in women and one of the most common complications experienced, which include itching with a thick vaginal discharge, burning during urination, redness and white patches at the sites of infection, and pain during sex [34].

Impotence

Impotence, or the inability to get or maintain an erection, may be caused by HIV damaging the nerves in the penis that control an erection (autonomic neuropathy). Similarly, anti-HIV drugs that cause neuropathy, such as ddC, ddI, and d4T, may cause numbness in the genital area, which can make it difficult to sustain an erection [50–53]. Protease inhibitors also have been reported to cause impotence, with some evidence suggesting that agents that contain ritonavir are particularly likely to cause sexual dysfunction [50–53].

Viagra (sidenafil) and Cialis (tadalafil), which are tablets used to treat impotence, work by increasing blood flow to the penis, making it more sensitive to touch. Viagra and Cialis should be taken with care by people using protease inhibitors, non-nucleoside reverse transcriptase inhibitors, ketoconazole, itraconazole, or erythromycin [50–53]. The dose of Viagra and Cialis should be reduced. For people taking ritonavir, however, it is recommended that Viagra not be used at all because of potential health risks. Similarly, recreational drug poppers must not be used with Viagra or Cialis under any circumstances.

Older interventions for impotence include the injection of alprostadil, a hormone produced by the prostate gland that alters the flow of blood in the penis. This can be done using Caverject, a tiny needle used to inject the penis with the hormone. It works quickly, and the effects can last for hours, although some men may find the process unappealing. The long-term effects are unknown and there is a limit of three injections a week, otherwise there is a risk of priapism, or persistent painful erection of the penis [50–53]. Alternatively, alprostadil comes as a pellet that is inserted into the urethra using an applicator. This application is known as Muse. A range of different implants is also available, but they need to be replaced as time passes. A semi-solid silicone implant can make the penis firmer, but not hard. Alternatively, a pocket can be created within the penis into which a silicone rod is inserted to form an erection. Vacuum pumps, including the Rapport pump, are also available.

It is not uncommon for HIV-positive women to experience early menopause as a result of abnormal production of the female hormones progesterone and estrogen [34]. Sexual dysfunction among women also can be caused by physical symptoms, such as vaginal dryness or thrush, pain, or severe premenstrual syndrome. Women can be offered hormone replacement therapy, although it should be monitored carefully [34].

Summary

The purpose of this article was to outline information about HIV, AIDS, and sexuality for nurses. There was a discussion of relationships, sexuality and sexual health, gender perceptions about sexuality, sexual needs and difficulties, and nursing assessment and intervention strategies. Overall, persons who are living with HIV/AIDS are sexual beings who desire to be loved and touched by others. Nursing is concerned with how people live their lives, and so it is fitting that nurses take a major health care role with people as they live with HIV/AIDS.

References

[1] US Surgeon General. Call to action to promote sexual health and responsible sexual behavior. Washington, DC: 2001.

[2] Boonstra H. Meeting the sexual and reproductive health needs of people living with HIV. Issues Brief (Alan Guttmacher Inst) 2006;6:1–4.

[3] CDC. Epidemiology of HIV/AIDS: United States, 2001–2005. MMWR Morb Mortal Wkly Rep 2006;55:589–92.

[4] Kiwana R, Garanganga E, Jagwe JGM. Human sexuality. In: Gwyther LA, Merriman A, Sebuyira LM, et al, editors. A clinical guide to supportive and palliative care for HIV/ AIDS in Sub-Saharan Africa. Alexandria (VA): Foundation for Hospices in Sub-Saharan Africa; 2006. p. 297–307.

[5] Anderson W. The needs of people living with HIV in the UK: a guide. National AIDS Trust. Jones and Palmer, Ltd; 2004. p. 10.

[6] Emlet CA. An examination of the social networks and social isolation in older and younger adults living with HIV/AIDS. Health Soc Work 2006;13:299–308.

[7] Lewis E. Afraid to say: the needs and views of people living with HIV/AIDS. London: National Children's Bureau and Strutton; 2004.

[8] Keegan A, Lambert S, Petrak J. Sex and relationships for HIV-positive women since HAART: a qualitative study. AIDS Patient Care STDS 2005;19:645–54.

[9] Martin JI. Self-esteem instability and its implications for HIV prevention among gay men. Health Soc Work 1997;22(4):264–73.

[10] Florence E, Schrooten W, Dreezen C, et al. Prevalence and factors associated with sexual dysfunction among HIV-positive women in Europe. AIDS Care 2004;16:550–7.

[11] Beckerman NL. Couples coping with discordant HIV status. AIDS Patient Care STDS 2002; 16(2):55–9.

[12] Summerside J, Davis M. Keeping it to ourselves: strategic directions in sexual health promotion and HIV prevention for people with HIV. London: Terrence Higgins Trust; 2004.

[13] Bogart LM, Collins RL, Kanouse DE, et al. Patterns and correlates of deliberate abstinence among men and women with HIV/AIDS. Am J Public Health 2006;96:1078–84.

[14] O'Leary A. Women at risk for HIV from a primary partner: balancing risk and intimacy. Annu Rev Sex Res 2000;11:191–234.

[15] Reynolds NR. Balancing disfigurement and fear of disease progression: patient perceptions of HIV body fat redistribution. AIDS Care 2006;18(7):663–73.

[16] Sharma A. Body image in older men with or at-risk for HIV infection. AIDS Care 2007; 19(2):235–41.

[17] Collazos J, Martinez E, Mayo J, et al. Sexual dysfunction in HIV-infected patients treated with highly active antiretroviral therapy. J Acquir Immune Defic Syndr 2002;31:322–6.

[18] World Health Organization. What constitutes sexual health, vol. 67, p. 3.

[19] Graham A. Sexual health. Br J Gen Pract 2004;54:382–7.

[20] Bell E, Van Beelen N. Exchange on HIV/AIDS, sexuality and gender. Amsterdam (The Netherlands): Royal Tropical Institute; 2006.

[21] Bova C, Durante A. Sexual functioning among HIV-infected women. AIDS Patient Care STDS 2003;17:75–83.

[22] Gurevich M, Mathieson CM, Bower J, et al. Disciplining bodies, desires, and subjectivities: sexuality and HIV-positive women. Fem Psychol 2007;17:9–38.

[23] CDC. HIV/AIDS among men who have sex with men: fact sheet. Washington, DC: Author; 2006.

[24] CDC. High-risk sexual behavior by HIV-positive men who have sex with men: 16 sites, United States, 2000–2002. MMWR Morb Mortal Wkly Rep 2004;53:891–4.

[25] Denning PH, Campsmith ML. Unprotected anal intercourse among HIV-positive men who have a steady male sex partner with negative or unknown HIV serostatus. Am J Public Health 2005;95:152–8.

[26] Woltski RJ, Parsons JT, Gomez CA. Prevention with HIV-seropositive men who have sex with men: lessons learned from the Seropositive Urban Men's Study (SUMS) and the Seropositive Urban Men's Intervention Trial (SUMIT). J Acquir Immune Defic Syndr 2004;37: S101–9.

[27] Mills TC, Stall R, Pollack L. Health-related characteristics of men who have sex with men: a comparison of those living in "gay ghettos" with those living elsewhere. Am J Public Health 2001;91:980–3.

[28] Diaz R. Latino gay men and psych-cultural barriers to AIDS prevention. In: Levin MP, Nardi PM, Gagnon JH, editors. Changing times: gay men and lesbian encounters HIV/ AIDS. Chicago: University of Chicago Press; 1997.

[29] Marin G, Marin BV. Research with Hispanic populations. Newbury Park (CA): Sage; 1991.

[30] Colegreco JP. Pathophysiology of HIV infection. In: Kirton C, editor. ANAC's core curriculum for HIV/AIDS nursing. 2nd edition. 2003. p. 22–8.

[31] Flaskerud JH, Ungvarski PJ. Overview and update of HIV disease. In: Ungvarski PJ, Flaskerud JH, editors. HIV/AIDS: a guide to primary care management. 4th edition. 1999. p. 1–25.

[32] Bennet JA. Epidemiology of HIV infection and AIDS. In: Kirton C, editor. ANAC's core curriculum for HIV/AIDS nursing. 2nd edition. 2003. p. 4–17.

[33] Burr CK, D'Orlando D. Perinatal transmission of HIV infection. In: Kirton C, editor. ANAC's core curriculum for HIV/AIDS nursing. 2nd edition. 2003. p. 242–6.

[34] Kurth A. Women, pregnant women, lesbians, and transgender/transsexual problems. In: Ungvarski PJ, Flaskerud JH, editors. HIV/AIDS: a guide to primary care management. 4th edition. 1999. p. 308–21.

[35] Krebs L. What should I say? Talking with patients about sexuality issues. Clin J Oncol Nurs 2006;10:313–5.

[36] Steinke EE. Intimacy needs and chronic illness: strategies for sexual counseling and self-management. J Gerontol Nurs 2005;31(5):40–50.

[37] CDC. A guide to taking a sexual history. Washington, DC: Author; 2005.

[38] Sharma A. Body image in middle-aged HIV-infected and uninfected women. AIDS Care 2006;18(8):998–1003.

[39] Huang JS. Body image in men with HIV. AIDS Patient Care STDS 2006;20:668–77.

[40] Neighbors CJ. Responses of male inmates to primary partner requests for condom use: effects of message content and domestic violence history. AIDS Educ Prev 2003;15: 93–108.

[41] Pulerwitz J. Relationship power, condom use and HIV risk among women in the USA. AIDS Care 2002;14:789–800.

[42] Lam AG. It takes two: the role of partner ethnicity and age characteristics on condom negotiations of heterosexual Chinese and Filipina American college women. AIDS Educ Prev 2006;18:68–80.

[43] Kordoutis PS. Heterosexual relationship characteristics, condom use and safe sex practices. AIDS Care 2000;12:767–82.

[44] Oette M, Junetzko P, Kroidl A, et al. Lipodystrophy syndrome and self-assessment of well-being and physical appearance in HIV-positive patients. AIDS Patient Care STDs 2000;16: 413–7.

[45] Dukers N, Stolte IG, Albrecht N, et al. The impact of experiencing lipodystrophy on the sexual behavior and well-being among HIV-infected homosexual men. AIDS 2001;15:812–3.

[46] Carter JA. Gender differences related to heterosexual condom use: the influence of negotiation styles. J Sex Marital Ther 1999;25:217–25.

[47] Soler H. Relationship dynamics, ethnicity and condom use among low-income women. Fam Plann Perspect 2000;32:82–8, 101.

[48] Tindall B. Sexual dysfunction in advanced HIV disease. AIDS Care 1994;6:105–7.

[49] Jones M. Psychosexual problems in people with HIV infection: controlled study of gay men and men with haemophilia. AIDS Care 1994;6:587–93.

[50] Schurmeyer TH, Mulier V, von zur Muhlen A, et al. Endocrine testicular function in HIV infected outpatients. Fur J Med Res 1997;2:275–81.

[51] Rabkin JG, Rabkin R, Wagner G. Testosterone replacement therapy in HIV illness. Gen Hosp Psychiatry 1995;17:37–42.

[52] Nusbaum MR, Hamilton C, Lenahan P. Chronic illness and sexual functioning. Am Fam Physician 2003;67:347–54, 357.

[53] Martinez E, Collazos J, Mayo J, et al. Sexual dysfunction with protease inhibitors. Lancet 1999;353:810–1.

[54] Schrooten W, Colebunders R, Youle M, et al. Sexual dysfunction associated with protease inhibitor containing highly active antiretroviral treatment. AIDS 2001;15:1019–23.

[55] Koenig LJ. Women, violence, and HIV: a critical evaluation with implications for HIV services. Matern Child Health J 2000;4:103–9.

[56] Schlitz MA, Sandfort ThGM. HIV-positive people, risk behaviour and sexual behaviour. Soc Sci Med 2000;50:1571–88.

ELSEVIER
SAUNDERS

NURSING
CLINICS
OF NORTH AMERICA

Nurs Clin N Am 42 (2007) 655–674

Chronic Illness Care for Lesbian, Gay, & Bisexual Individuals

Suzanne L. Dibble, DNSc, RN[a],*,
Michele J. Eliason, PhD, RN[b],
Mats A.D. Christiansen, MNSc, RN[c,d]

[a]Institute for Health & Aging, School of Nursing, University
of California, San Francisco, San Francisco, CA, USA
[b]Health Education, San Francisco State University, San Francisco, CA, USA
[c]Family Health Care Nursing, University of California, San Francisco,
San Francisco, USA
[d]Division of Nursing, Department of Neurobiology, Care Sciences
and Society Karolinska Institutet, Huddinge, Sweden

In every part of the United States, in every hospital, in every long-term care facility, in every outpatient clinic, in every school and community, and in every practice, nurses are caring for lesbian, gay, and bisexual (LGB) clients. In the 2000 census, same-sex unmarried partners were present in 99.3% of all counties in the United States [1]. Results from the National Health and Social Life Survey indicated that at least 1.51% of the population identifies itself as openly LGB [2]. To put this number in perspective, this percentage is more than the percentage of the population who are Presbyterian (1.3%); Jewish (1.3%); American Indian/Alaskan native (0.9%); or vegan (0.2%). See *www.adherents.com/adh_dem.html* for additional information.

LGB clients often are an invisible subgroup among those who are chronically ill. Most, especially older LGB people, have experienced antihomosexual prejudice, and many have experienced threats or violence, sometimes from health care providers [3,4]. Thus, secrecy was and is important for many LGB individuals, especially among older generations. Two very common assumptions have posed barriers to quality care of LGB patients. First, the assumption by nurses that all clients are heterosexual has a negative impact on potentially supportive interactions with LGB clients by virtually

---

* Corresponding author.
E-mail addresses: sue.dibble@ucsf.edu; sue.dibble@gmail.com (S.L. Dibble).

rendering them invisible. A second assumption by nurses that the world contains only two genders (male or female) also negatively affects their interactions with LGB patients who often violate societal norms for their gender (it also significantly affects intersex and transgender patients, some of whom are also LGB).

Nurses caring for LGB clients may know the sexual orientation or gender identity of their clients, but often they may not. Learning how to obtain information and how to use it is the focus of this chapter. The Awareness, Sensitivity, and Knowledge (ASK™) framework can be used to obtain and apply the essential information needed to provide culturally appropriate nursing care [5]. We must be *aware* of our own beliefs and biases about LGB people—heterosexism, the belief that heterosexuality is the only normal option for relationships—is deeply engrained and taken for granted. We need *sensitivity* in our approach to care and *knowledge* to inform our practice [5]. In the remainder of this chapter, we discuss (1) important definitions that describe LGB lives, (2) disclosure of sexual identities, (3) risk factors and data on chronic illness issues for LGB patients, and (4) how to conduct vital assessments about sexuality.

Definitions

Sexual orientation is an enduring emotional, romantic, sexual, or affectional attraction toward others. It is easily distinguished from other components of sexuality including biological sex, gender identity (the psychological sense of being male or female), and the social gender role (adherence to cultural norms for feminine and masculine behavior). Sexual orientation exists along a continuum that ranges from exclusive heterosexuality to exclusive homosexuality and includes various forms of bisexuality. Bisexual persons can experience sexual, emotional, and affectional attraction to both their own sex and the opposite sex [6].

Persons with a same-sex orientation often are referred to as gay (both men and some women) or as lesbian (women only). Younger individuals may call themselves "queer"; however, some older LGB individuals consider this word offensive. Many LGB individuals may also consider the word "homosexual" to be an insult. It is safest for nurses to use the words that patients use to describe themselves or use the more generic "sexual orientation." Sexual orientations are the public fact about who people are attracted to and say nothing about a person's private sexual behaviors. It is important to remember that behaviors may not be congruent with one's sexual orientation—that is, a woman who identifies as a lesbian may have recent or past sexual experiences with men, and a self-identified heterosexual woman may have considerable same-sex experience. In this chapter, we combine bisexual women with lesbians and bisexual men with gay men for most of our discussions, because there is insufficient evidence to be more specific. However, it is likely that experiences with health care differ by many social identities, including race/ethnicity, social standing, education, sex, gender, and sexual orientation, so we recognize that we are glossing over potentially important differences (Box 1).

It is also important to note that the definitions of sex/gender and sexuality have developed out of white, middle class value and belief systems and that those from other cultural groups may use different terms (For instance *mahu* in French Polynesia; *hijras* in India and Pakistan; *fa'afafin* in Samoa; or *tomboi*, in the Philippines) and have different understandings about sex/gender and sexuality [10,11]. Another example is the term "two spirit" which is used to define Native American people's sexual identities; this

---

Box 1. Gender clarification

The term "transgender" is used to describe people whose gender identity is not congruent with their sex as assigned at their birth. A male-to-female transgender individual is a transgender woman ("trans woman") and a female-to-male transgender individual is a transgender man ("trans man"). There are some individuals in the transgender community who do not identify as either male or female, but "gender queer." Transitioning, the process that many transgender people undergo to bring their outward gender expression into alignment with their gender identity, can involve medical treatments such as hormonal therapy, cosmetic procedures, and genital surgery [7,8]. There are also gender nonconforming people who do not identify as transgender and may express their individuality in dress, in behaviors, and/or speech (See Skidmore, Linsenmeier, & Bailey [9] for more details).

"Intersex" is a general term used for a number of conditions in which a person has reproductive or sexual anatomy that does not fit the typical definitions of female or male. A person might be born appearing to be female on the outside but having mostly male-typical anatomy on the inside. Or a person may be born with genitals that seem to be in-between the usual male and female types—for example, a girl may be born with a noticeably large clitoris or lacking a vaginal opening, or a boy may be born with a notably small penis, or with a scrotum that is divided like a labia. See www.isna.org/faq/what_is_intersex for more information. Transgender and intersex individuals may have lesbian, gay, bisexual, or heterosexual orientations.

Suggested readings: Meyer IH, Northridge M, eds. The health of sexual minorities: Public health perspectives on lesbian, gay, bisexual, and transgender populations. New York: Springer; 2007.

term does not equate to lesbian, gay, bisexual, transgender, or intersex, but denotes a greater level of sexual and gender fluidity that is common to many Native American groups [12,13]. Information about transgender and intersex persons are very complex and beyond the scope of this chapter.

The term "family" is frequently used among LGB individuals to denote something broader than family of origin— an affinity circle that has significant meaning for those who participate in it. Many LGB individuals have been rejected by their families of origin. The most commonly used term applied to LGB networks is "family of choice" [14]. This family is composed of the people, usually the partner and friends, who share, support, and care for the LGB individual. Often included in these networks are ex-lovers and/or ex-spouses. Many LGB families fear exclusion and discrimination from health care providers and institutions. Most hospitals and clinics use the narrow definitions of family that are sanctioned by laws in most states: the only legitimate adult relationships are those between one man and one woman and the offspring of those unions, parents, or siblings, and they may exclude LGB family members from critical health care decisions and settings if the family does not fit legal definitions. As an example, one respondent told this story: "It was real important to me that Shannon, my partner, was the person that the doctor recognized as my primary relationship and gave her the information...We just recently had a friend, an older woman, who went through a terrible loss of her long-time partner. After her partner died on the operating table, the doctor left the friend in the waiting room while he told the biological family— not the friend—that her partner had died. To compound this error, the biological family went home without telling the friend about the death of her partner" [15].

LGB family forms are varied and can include couples in civil unions, domestic partnerships, or legally unrecognized long-term, committed relationships; open relationships; or group families (for example, a lesbian couple and a gay couple conceive and raise children together). Children can come into the family from previous heterosexual relationships, alternative insemination procedures, adoption, and coparenting.

Disclosure: "outness" or secrecy?

Sexual and gender identities are not always visible differences and therefore require disclosure to health care providers. There are a number of reasons why LGB people might not disclose their sexuality or gender identity to a health care provider. For example, Boehmer and Case [16] interviewed 39 lesbian and bisexual women with a diagnosis of breast cancer and found that 72% had disclosed their sexuality to their health care provider (HCP). Those who disclosed said they did so because the environment seemed safe and/or they had done preparatory work in researching the HCP before scheduling an appointment. Most of them had disclosed in the context of written or verbal questions about marital status, stating that their partner was female or bringing a partner to appointments. Women who chose not to disclose did so because of fear of homophobic reactions, being single, or holding a belief that one's sexual orientation is private (see also, Hitchcock and Wilson [17]; Stevens [4]). A woman in treatment for breast cancer remarked about her decision whether or not to disclose to the surgeon: "And having to worry [that] is she homophobic and [wonder] will she take another snip out that she is not supposed to?" [16].

LGB people of color may be even less likely than white LGB people to disclose their sexuality to a HCP because of cultural norms about the privacy of sexuality [18–21], religious beliefs [22], not relating to the gay male culture [23], or family obligations related to marriage and family [24]. There may be even greater mistrust of health care providers and systems among LGB people of color than white LGB people because of historical abuses [25–27].

Disclosure varies by generation, gender, ethnicity, couple status, and reason for seeking care. Eliason and Schope [28] studied disclosure to health care providers in a sample of mostly white, well-educated lesbian, gay, and bisexual respondents. Disclosure was defined as not merely out or not out to health care provider, but disclosure was seen as active (patients told the HCP of their sexuality) or passive (patients wore a t-shirt or button proclaiming their sexuality or told the HCP a partner's name). Nondisclosure could also be active (lying) or passive (saying nothing). Table 1 illustrates some of the data from this study divided by gender, showing that women were more likely to actively disclose and were also more likely to have a will and power of attorney for health care than male respondents. Very few respondents had power of attorney for health care, a troubling finding in this highly educated sample.

Several studies have indicated that LGB patients would prefer that their HCP ask them directly about their sexuality, either in written or oral assessments. Lucas [29] reported that 64% of lesbians wanted the HCP to ask directly, or as one respondent in another study put it: "One doctor I went to, actually, on the questionnaire, optional information was 'Were you

Table 1
LGB respondents' strategies and experiences with health care providers

Characteristic	Lesbian and bisexual women (n = 47)	Gay and bisexual men (n = 41)
Actively disclosed sexuality to HCP in the most recent visit	43%	29%
Passively avoided discussion of sexuality and HCP did not ask	34%	42%
Actively lied about sexuality	0	2%
Had a will	32%	22%
Had durable power of attorney for health care	6%	2%

heterosexual, lesbian, or gay or bisexual?' And that was wonderful. I could just tell him and they wouldn't be asking if they weren't open and aware" [30]. A recent survey of LGB youth found that 64% preferred that physicians "just ask me" about their sexual identity [31]. Situations in which disclosure might be unlikely could include older LGBs who grew up in a more restrictive, homophobic environment than that of today; LGBs of color who have more to lose by disclosing; LGBs in the military for whom "don't tell" is a mandate; and situations in which sexuality is not considered to be relevant, such as being treated in an emergency room for a minor injury.

Risk factors for chronic illness

There is very little research on the prevalence of chronic illnesses among LGB people; however, there are several reasons why LGB people may experience a greater frequency of many chronic disorders. Many of these are related to stigma. Sexual stigma is "society's shared belief system through which homosexuality is denigrated, discredited, and constructed as invalid relative to heterosexuality" [32]. For many LGB people, sexual stigma is internalized as a strong sense of shame, guilt, or self-hatred [33–35]. This internalization is variously referred to in the literature as internalized homophobia, oppression, stigma, or heterosexism. Stigma has a number of effects, including:

1. *Minority stress*: LGB people deal with chronic levels of daily stress related to stigma. The greater the number of stigmatized identities, the higher the level of stress, which suggests that LGB people of color may have even higher rates of stress and stress-related disorders than white LGBs [36]. Considerable research has found the link between racism and physical and mental health disorders (eg, Williams and colleagues [37]), but less research has examined the effects of negative attitudes about LGB people on their health and well-being. Most of the existing research has focused on sexual risk-taking behavior [27,38,39], substance abuse [40,41], and mental illness [42]. Stress-related mental health problems such as depression have also been found to have associated physical health consequences [43–45].

2. *Higher rates of substance abuse* [46], especially smoking [47], may be associated with higher levels of chronic diseases and cancers. It is possible that excessive rates of chronic illnesses are largely caused by the higher rates of smoking, alcohol use, and drug abuse among the LGB communities. See Fig. 1 which describes a conceptual model of chronic illness that includes sexual orientation as a predictor variable.

3. *Discrimination affects access to care*: discrimination in the workplace means that more LGB people may work in lower paying jobs without benefits or need to hide their sexuality and relationships on the job; discrimination related to relationships means that more LGB people in

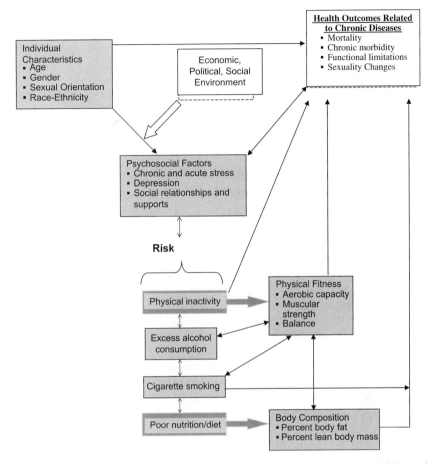

Fig. 1. Conceptual framework of determinants of disease disparities between lesbian and heterosexual women (Pruitt and Dibble, personal communication, 2005).

committed relationships lack health insurance benefits that married heterosexual couples have. Heck and colleagues [48] reported that women in same-sex relationships were significantly less likely than women in opposite-sex relationships to have health insurance, to have seen a medical provider in the last year, or to have a regular health care provider. Men in same-sex relationships were similar to heterosexual men on these variables.

4. *Experiences or fear of discrimination* by health care systems and providers means that many **LGBT** people do not get preventative care or delay accessing care until conditions have progressed [26,49–51]. For example, several studies have found that lesbians are less likely than heterosexual women to get regular pap tests and breast examinations [52,53].

Research information about chronic conditions within the lesbian and gay communities is sparse or nonexistent except that relating to human immunodeficiency virus (HIV) or breast cancer. Many researchers in the United States just do not include the questions about sexual orientation in studies of chronic illness. In a recent Dutch study, Bakker and colleagues [54] showed that rates of reporting of at least one chronic illness were higher among the adult LGB population than among heterosexuals. For women, the rates of at least one chronic illness were 70% for heterosexual women, 75% for bisexuals, and 80% for lesbians. For men, those reporting at least one chronic illness were 59% of heterosexuals, 40% of bisexuals, and 70% of gay men. The types of chronic illness were not reported. Our best guess is that LGB people experience many chronic illnesses at the same rate as the general population but may be at higher risk for certain chronic illnesses.

The leading cause of death in the United States is cardiovascular disease (CVD); therefore, it is likely that it is the leading cause of death for LGB people. Higher rates of CVD than in the general population are expected in LGBs because of the higher rates of smoking, alcohol and drug use, and obesity in women [55,56]. In a recent study in Switzerland, Wang and his colleagues [57] reported that gay men were significantly less likely to be overweight than their heterosexual counterparts; however, they reported significantly more and severe physical symptoms and short-term disabilities. The common risk factors for chronic diseases—high cholesterol, high blood pressure, high glucose, and smoking—were all significantly higher for gay men when compared with heterosexual men even after adjustment for differences in sociodemographic characteristics and health behaviors.

Lung and breast cancer are the most common cancers in women, and lesbian/bisexual women may have higher risk factors for both of these. With regard to lung cancer, more lesbian/bisexual women smoke than heterosexual women, and it is quite likely that more nonsmoking lesbian/bisexual women live with a smoking partner than do heterosexual women, increasing their risk for exposure to second- and third-hand smoke. Risk factors for breast cancer include nulliparity, smoking and alcohol use, and obesity, all of which are more common among most lesbian communities [58,59]. Research pertaining to physical activity levels in heterosexual and lesbian women suggests there was no difference in the prevalence of sedentary behavior between lesbians and a national probability sample of women in the United States [60]. However, this same study reported that when lesbians were active, they were more likely than the general population of women to engage in vigorous physical activity.

Lung cancer is not the only respiratory problem of LGB individuals. Heck and Jacobson [48] examined lifetime and current asthma diagnoses among persons in same-sex relationships (SSRs) using data from the pooled 1997–2004 National Health Interview Surveys. They found that 13.5% of gay men and 14.3% of lesbians reported a lifetime diagnosis of asthma, compared with 7.6% and 10.2% of respondents in opposite-sex relationships. Those in SSRs may be at higher risk for asthma because of a spectrum of risk factors including higher rates of smoking; stress; and, among women, obesity [48]. After reviewing www.pubmed.gov for studies of COPD among LGB people, no studies have yet to be reported. We would presume that the rates would be increased in LGBs because of the higher rates of smoking and asthma.

Men with HIV/acquired immunodeficiency syndrome (AIDS) are also more prone to lymphoma [61], anal dysplasias as well as carcinoma [62], and certain sarcomas (Kaposi's in particular [63]). Since first described in the literature in 1981, the AIDS epidemic in the United States has had devastating effects on people from all subsets of the population but has hit marginalized groups the hardest. Men who have sex with men still comprise the largest category of those infected, with men of color disproportionately represented [64]. Mortality has decreased with the advent of new antiretroviral treatments, making HIV infection more like other chronic illnesses, but there are consequences associated with the newer treatments. These consequences include drug side effects that affect body image and sexuality, the greater chance of transmitting the virus to partners because of longer life span (but where successful treatments are believed to decrease the risk of transmission because of lowered viral loads), and issues of access to treatment because of the high cost. Sexual dysfunctions related to HIV have been attributed to the antiretroviral treatment, pathophysiologic factors related to the disease from neuropathy, and also psychological factors. And there can of course be a combination of factors causing the dysfunction [65,66]. A longer and healthier life as an infected person also raises issues of disclosure of the seropositivity to partners and the ability to engage in and sustain harm-reducing behaviors.

Prostate cancer is another common cancer that can affect gay and bisexual male patients. It has been noted that few of the studies regarding prostate cancer have included gay men. Unfortunately, most of the patient information has been created for heterosexual men in their relationships with women [67] and, therefore, may not be relevant to men who have sex with men. For prostate cancer, and many other surgical procedures in the pelvic cavity (eg, colorectal cancer and some orthopedic surgery), there are risks for problems with erectile function.

Treatments for erectile dysfunction (ED) like sildenafil, tadalafil and vardenafil, have become more commonly used. However, many gay men combine ED drugs with recreational drugs in an attempt to enhance sexual experiences [68]. This combination of substances has been shown to relate to riskier sexual behavior in the form of a larger number of sexual partners and unprotected intercourse [69–71]. In some groups of gay men, the use of poppers (amyl nitrite) in sexual practices increases risk because ED drugs and poppers interact and can cause lethal hypotension. There are also reports of dangerous interactions of ED drugs when combined with methamphetamine and other recreational drugs [66].

Treatment issues related to chronic illness care for lesbian, gay, and bisexual patients

This section reviews some treatment issues related to sexual identity and chronic illness care, including creating a welcoming environment, issues for families and partners, managing inappropriate comments and behaviors, treatment options, and determining the relevance of sexual identity to care.

Creating a welcoming health care environment

Ways to show that a health care setting is inclusive and welcoming to LGB individuals can include visual markers such as posters that depict same-sex couples, forms that are inclusive, brochures and patient pamphlets that deal with LGB issues and prominently displayed human rights policies, and training of all employees in inclusiveness (receptionists, housekeepers, dietary workers, technicians). The website for the Gay and Lesbian Medical Association has a pamphlet on creating a welcoming environment (www.glma.org). Inclusive language is a key component to a welcoming environment and is discussed in detail in the section on assessment. Finding a supportive environment for LGBs with chronic illnesses may be particularly challenging when identifying support groups. Support groups are enormously helpful for many people in sharing their experiences and learning from others how to cope with living with a chronic illness. If the group facilitator or group members are uncomfortable with the LGB member, the LGB person is unlikely to benefit from attending the group. A respondent in a study of lesbians with disabilities had this to say: "Firstly [I want people to know]…that we exist…Too often people don't think of people with disabilities as sexual beings at all—or if they do, our sexuality is thought of as a problem…Disability sets you apart from other queer women. Sexuality sets you apart from other women with disabilities. It's easy to feel very, very isolated" [72]. Nurses should not only be aware of the inclusivity of their own clinic/hospital/practice, but also of any referral sources that the health care agency uses for support services for their patients. This issue can be critical in settings in which group treatments are the standard, such as substance abuse treatment settings—the LGB client may have to face negative reactions or lack of understanding from counselors and other clients [73].

Managing inappropriate comments/behaviors

LGB people often have experienced negative comments from health care providers. Just as you would not tolerate a racist comment from a colleague, nurses need to intervene when antigay comments and "jokes" occur in the workplace. That intervention could be a comment to the "joker" or reporting the individual. These types of comments are distressing at any time to your LGB coworkers, but imagine that you are a patient and feeling vulnerable and hear "all she needs is a good sex (he really used the 'f' word) with a man" as one of the authors (Dibble) heard the chief resident say on rounds outside her door. The subsequent laughter from the nurses and physicians was the worst. As one respondent in Stevens and Halls research said, "it's like putting your life in someone's hands who really hates you." [74]. Here are a few other examples of experiences of LGB people:

"I have had a female doctor say she was fine with it and then try to coerce me into saying sexual identity is purely a choice. My worst experience, the doctor lectured me on the Bible and changed her diagnosis (gay male, age 28)" [28].

"He asked if I was married. When I said, 'No, I live with my lesbian lover,' he was quite embarrassed. Then he told me not to be embarrassed" [75].

"As soon as I said I was a lesbian, the nurses started giving me disgusting looks. They were nasty to my partner. They rough-housed me. They were not gentle like they would be to a straight woman. They treated me like I was 'one of those' like they might catch something" [74].

Treatment of partners and family of choice

Partners often are treated poorly in health care settings, adding additional stress to the situation. As one woman said about her partner's hospitalization:

In my experience as both patient and close relative, it's been worse to be the relative—as a patient, they pretty much have to take care of me, but as a relative they can ignore me—like my being there makes the patient homosexual—if I weren't there, she would just be another patient in the lot. But since she had me with her—she suddenly became something else— and it's probably easier to just close your eyes and pretend I'm not there— but I can really only interpret it as if they didn't accept that we had a homosexual relationship—they would much rather talk to our parents, even though we are adults (woman, 30 years old)" [76].

Treatment options

Complementary and alternative medicines (CAM) are used by most non–chronically ill lesbians [77]. In fact, these researchers reported that the predictors of CAM use included a lesbian sexual orientation, less health-related worry, and perceived discrimination in health care settings. In another study of those with HIV, CAM use was higher for people who were gay/lesbian, had incomes above $40,000, lived in the Northeast and West, were depressed, and wanted more information about and more decision-making involvement in their care [78]. Because CAM use is so widespread among the LGB communities, the nurse must assess the potential interaction of the CAM therapies, especially herbs and supplements, on the treatment plan for an individual. Many clinical pharmacists can assist with this process.

Relevance of sexual identity to care

Sexuality may or may not be directly relevant to the patient's care, but it is likely that there often will be times when it is relevant. LGB patients will respond to the same medications, the same diet and exercise plans, and the same surgical or physical procedures as heterosexual patients, but their adjustment or coping with the chronic illness might be significantly affected by sexual orientation. For example, there is a high value placed on self-reliance in the LGB community, thus, a debilitating or disabling chronic illness may make the LGB person feel alienated from LGB peers or feel a greater sense of shame or guilt about their limitations [72]. Many clients feel a need to maintain control over who sees them unclothed; therefore, you should ask a patient's permission first before inviting a colleague or student nurse into the room when the patient is unclothed or will be unclothed. This is particularly true for transgender and intersex clients. It is important to assess how sexuality might affect chronic illness care and adaptation for each unique individual.

Sexuality and chronic illness: assessment issues

Sexual disorders and anxieties about sexuality are very common in patients with chronic illnesses, and these sexual problems have both physiologic and psychological origins [79,80]. Many nurses believe that sexuality assessment, evaluation, and counseling are a part of their professional role; however, nurses do not necessarily integrate this awareness into their patient care. Discomfort, embarrassment, or strongly held beliefs about the nurse's role in discussing sexuality with patients can act as barriers to responding to these patient concerns [81]. This discomfort is compounded when there is not congruence between the sexual orientation of the nurse and the client, especially if the nurse is heterosexual and brought up to believe that heterosexuality is the only appropriate and proper sexual orientation. Other barriers to completing a proper assessment of sexual health in patients in general include: (1) the nurses' perceptions that patients do not expect nurses to address their sexuality concerns; (2) lack of knowledge and confidence in addressing sexuality; and (3) failure to make time to discuss patient sexuality concerns [82]. We will discuss assessment of sexual health from two perspectives. The first section addresses sexual identities and family issues, and the final section addresses the assessment of specific sexual practices or behaviors.

Assessing sexual and gender identities

Assessment generally includes two formats for acquiring information from clients: written forms and oral interactions (intakes, histories, or assessments). Written forms can be made more inclusive by adding a few simple questions or altering existing ones to provide more options or use different language. For the assessment of sex/gender, adding an option for other (or if there is sufficiently large population of transgender and intersex clients in the practice, adding these options) is usually sufficient. Sexuality can be assessed by asking whether clients identify as heterosexual, gay, lesbian, bisexual, questioning, not sure/don't know, or other. A follow-up question can ask if the client wants this information noted on their medical record. Sexual behavior can be assessed by asking whether the client has had sex with exclusively men, mostly men, both men and women, mostly women, or exclusively women—this should be tied to some timeframe that makes the most sense for the setting, and can include lifetime, past year, or past month. Finally, in place of or in addition to questions about marital status (legal relationships—in states in which domestic partnerships or civil unions are possible, these should be included), a question about relationship status can include much broader categories such as single, married, committed relationship, separated, divorced, and other. There should also be a question on all written intake forms about legal documents that specify power of attorney for health care. If the client indicates they do not have such a document, a follow-up question can ask if they would like information on obtaining durable power of attorney. Finally, there should be a question such as "who do you want involved in your health care planning and decision making?"

The oral assessment is the best place to facilitate a good nurse–patient relationship. It is important not to make assumptions about the identity, beliefs, concerns, behaviors, or sexual orientation of any clients, but particularly those who are transgender, intersex, or do not adhere to cultural norms for feminine and masculine behavior. It can be uncomfortable to be confused about someone's gender and awkward to ask someone about their gender. If you are unsure about a person's gender identity or how they wish to be addressed, ask politely for clarification. If you let the person know that you are only trying to be respectful, your question will usually be appreciated. For instance, you can ask, "How would you like to be addressed?" "What name would you like to be called?" "Which pronoun is appropriate?" If the motivation for asking the question is only your own curiosity and is unrelated to care, it is inappropriate and can quickly create distance between you and the client and can be perceived as discrimination by the client. Just as you would not needlessly disclose a person's HIV status, a person's gender identity or sexual orientation is not an item for gossip. If disclosure is relevant to care, use discretion and inform the patient to whom you have disclosed their information whenever possible.

For LGB individuals with chronic illnesses, there are several important issues that the nurses should address. "What name do you like to be called?" Showing respect for your patient is the primary goal. Automatically using someone's first name is absolutely inappropriate unless directed to by the patient—err on the side of formality, not familiarity. The nurse is not a friend of the patient, but a source of information and care. By keeping the contact more formal, the nurse indicates professional behavior and gives the request for all information, including information about the patient's sexuality, more credibility. This outward sign of professionalism denotes that the nurse will handle all of the patient's private information appropriately and with respect.

Determining the relationship of the patient to important others is the next phase of the assessment process. There are multiple ways to do this. Asking if the patient is married is inappropriate unless you live in Massachusetts where same sex marriage is legal. Except in Massachusetts, this question indicates a presumption of heterosexuality and may shut down communication with your lesbian and gay clients. A better approach would be to start the assessment with, "Do you have a partner or significant others?" If the patient responds yes, then ask, "Do you want them with us for our discussion?" Although this seems obvious that the partner or significant other would be welcome, this is not the perception of most LGB clients. Your invitation tells the patient that you are open and willing to engage with the patient's family no matter how they define "family."

Once the relationship status has been identified, it is very important that you determine whether a durable power of attorney for health care has been completed. After an introduction about the importance of backup plans for those with (name their chronic illness), the question that should be asked is "Who do you want to speak for you if you cannot?" When the patient answers a name or names, then ask "Is this in writing and could we get a copy for our record?" Completing legal documents to protect relationships is very important for LGB people in same-sex relationships In most states, in the absence of written directions, health care professionals will turn to blood relatives to make decisions. This is true no matter how long LGB clients may have been with their partners and regardless of whether there is a good relationship or even any relationship with the blood relatives. The only exceptions are in states with laws that protect same-sex relationships. At the time of this writing, those included same-sex married spouses in Massachusetts, registered domestic partners in California and Maine, civil union spouses in Connecticut, New Jersey, and Vermont, and reciprocal beneficiaries in Hawaii. Even if your client lives in one of the states listed above and is in a legally recognized relationship, all couples and singles are encouraged to leave written instructions in the event that they become ill or incapacitated while in another state that refuses to honor the relationship. Everyone should carry copies of their authorizations at all times. See www.nclrights. org/publications/lifelines1005.htm for information that you can share with your clients. No one likes to think about being unable to make their own health care decisions, and LGB people are no exception. In a recent study of 1000 LGB baby boomers, more than one half (51%) have yet to complete wills or living wills spelling out their long-term care and end-of-life wishes [83]. Thus, one very important role for the nurse caring for these individuals is to help them understand the importance of having these documents today, not next week, next month, or next year.

Now that you have established a respectful, knowledgeable relationship with your clients, you can now begin to explore the impact of their chronic illness(es) in their lives. Because patients are the experts regarding their lives, the next question to ask is, "Would you please give me a brief history about your (name the chronic condition)." Amidst the discussion of the limitations caused by the disease or its treatment, you might ask "Has your (name the chronic condition) or the drugs used to treat it gotten in the way with your ability to make love or have sex? Please do not ask the question if you are not prepared to help. Common ways that chronic illnesses may affect sexual functioning include diminished sexual desire, erectile dysfunction, shame about the body (negative body image), reduced sensation, and the need to alter sexual positions or activities because of physical limitations.

Assessing sexual practices/behaviors

In preparing to problem solve with lesbian and gay patients around issues of sexuality and chronic illness, nurses must understand and be comfortable with discussing the components of sexual activities for lesbians and gay men. Considering that most nurses are uncomfortable talking about sexual practices even with their heterosexual patients, this is a challenge to nurses to develop a new skill set. In general, there are an infinite number of sexual practices of which any individual, couple, or group can engage, and these are not generally defined by one's sexual identity. These sexual behaviors can be solo (masturbation, use of sex toys, or fantasies) or interactive as part of a couple or a group. They may involve penetration (vaginal, oral, anal) or not; they can be physically intensive and exhausting or not. There are also a diverse array of consensual sexual practices that may include sexual roleplay and fetishes. The types of sexual behaviors that any patient might engage in are influenced by age, education, cultural norms, religion, level of comfort with one's own body and physical functioning, experiences of sexual abuse and traumas, partner's wishes, and comfort level with one's sexual identity, among a host of others. In fact, these factors are probably more predictive of sexual practice than one's sexual orientation.

Physical relationships for both genders can begin with various forms of nonpenetrative practices such as fondling, caressing, rubbing, and kissing. Penetrative practices can include manual, oral, vaginal, or anal insertive sex using body parts or sex toys. As with heterosexual couples, lesbian and gay couples can be inventive in their sexual practices. The *Whole Lesbian Sex Book* [84] offers a general compendium of basic information, techniques, advice, and support on the subject of lesbian sexual activities. Gay men's sexual activities are covered in *The Joy of Gay Sex* [85]. These books may be helpful to both you and your patients who need to alter their sexual practices in suggesting the wide range of ways that people can be intimate or sexual with each other or by themselves.

Summary

To summarize using the ASKmodel [5], we have attempted to raise awareness of LGB people's lives and health by providing basic definitions of sexual orientation and gender, describing LGB family forms, and reviewing the risk factors for chronic illness. Although data are limited, it appears that LGB people have more risk factors, and therefore, would be expected to experience higher rates of chronic illnesses than heterosexual people. This chapter has also focused on sensitivity to LGB people via the discussion of the impact of sexual stigma on health and well-being and sharing some of the bad experiences LGB people have had with health care workers and institutions. Finally, we have addressed knowledge deficits by providing a review of the literature, although limited, on chronic illness among LGB people, and by providing concrete suggestions for making assessments more inclusive of all clients' needs. Assessing for factors related to sexuality and gender need to become a routine part of the health care assessment process for all clients, and nurses are the ideal people to collect this information.

References

[1] Smith D, Gates GJ. Gay and lesbian families in the United States: same-sex unmarried partner households. A Preliminary Analysis of 2000 United States Census Data. Human Rights Campaign; 2001. Available at: http://www.urban.org/url.cfm?ID=1000491.

[2] Laumann EO. The social organization of sexuality: sexual practices in the United States. Chicago (IL): University of Chicago Press; 1994.

[3] Schatz B, O'Hanlan K. Anti-gay discrimination in medicine: results of a national survey of lesbian, gay, and bisexual physicians. San Francisco CA: American Association for Human Rights; 1994.

[4] Stevens PE. Protective strategies of lesbian clients in health care environments. Res Nurs Health 1994;17(3):217–29.

[5] Lipson JG, Dibble SL. Providing culturally appropriate health care. In: Lipson JG, Dibble SL, editors. Culture & clinical care. San Francisco (CA): UCSF Nursing Press; 2005. p. xi–xviii.

[6] APA Help Center. Sexual orientation and homosexuality. Available at: http://www.apahelpcenter.org/articles/article.php?id=31. Accessed March 15, 2007.

[7] Lawrence AA. Transgender health concerns. In: Meyer IH, Northridge M, editors. The health of sexual minorities: public health perspectives on lesbian, gay, bisexual, and transgender populations. New York: Springer; 2007. p. 473–505.

[8] Lombardi E. Public health and transpeople: barriers to care and strategies to improve treatment. In: Meyer IH, Northridge M, editors. The health of sexual minorities: public health perspectives on lesbian, gay, bisexual, and transgender populations. New York: Springer; 2007. p. 607–38.

[9] Skidmore WC, Linsenmeier JA, Bailey JM. Gender nonconformity and psychological distress in lesbians and gay men. Arch Sex Behav 2006;35(6):685–97.

[10] Herdt GH. Third sex, third gender: beyond sexual dimorphism in culture and history. New York: Zone Books; 1994.

[11] Roscoe W. Changing ones: third and fourth genders in Native North America. 1st edition. New York: St. Martin's Press; 1998.

[12] Fieland K, Walters K, Simoni J. Determinants of health among two-spirit American Indians and Alaska natives. In: Meyer IH, Northridge M, editors. The health of sexual minorities: public health perspectives on lesbian, gay, bisexual, and transgender populations. New York: Springer; 2007. p. 268–300.

[13] Tafoya T, Rowell R. Counseling gay and lesbian Native Americans. In: Shernoff M, Scott W, editors. The sourcebook on lesbian/gay health care. Washington DC: National Lesbian and Gay Health Foundation; 1988. p. 63–7.

[14] Weston K. Families we choose: lesbians, gays, and kinship. New York: Columbia University Press; 1991.

[15] Saulnier CF. Deciding who to see: lesbians discuss their preferences in health and mental health care providers. Soc Work 2002;47(4):355–65.

[16] Boehmer U, Case P. Physicians don't ask, sometimes patients tell: disclosure of sexual orientation among women with breast carcinoma. Cancer 2004;101(8):1882–9.

[17] Hitchcock JM, Wilson HS. Personal risking: lesbian self-disclosure of sexual orientation to professional health care providers. Nurs Res 1992;41(3):178–83.

[18] Chng CL, Wong FY, Park RJ, et al. A model for understanding sexual health among Asian American/Pacific Islander men who have sex with men (MSM) in the United States. AIDS Educ Prev 2003;15(1 Suppl A):21–38.

[19] Díaz RM. Latino gay men and HIV: culture, sexuality, and risk behavior. New York: Routledge; 1998.

[20] Dowd SA. Therapists on the frontline: psychotherapy with gay men in the age of AIDS. In: Caldwell S, Burnham R, Forstein M, editors. Therapists on the frontline: psychotherapy with gay men in the age of AIDS. Washington, DC: American Psychiatric Press; 1994. p. 319–38.

[21] Gomez C, Marin BV. Barriers to HIV prevention strategies for women. J Sex Res 1996;33: 355–62.

[22] Woodyard JL, Peterson JL, Stokes JP. "Let us go into the house of the Lord": participation in African American churches among young African American men who have sex with men. J Pastoral Care 2000;54(4):451–60.

[23] Wolitski RJ, Jones KT, Wasserman JL, et al. Self-identification as "down low" among men who have sex with men (MSM) from 12 US cities. AIDS Behav 2006;10(5): 519–29.

[24] Morales ES. HIV infection and Hispanic gay and bisexual men. Hisp J Behav Sci 1990;12: 212–22.

[25] Battle J, Crum M. Black LGB health and wellbeing. In: Meyer IH, Northridge M, editors. The health of sexual minorities: public health perspectives on lesbian, gay, bisexual, and transgender populations. New York: Springer; 2007. p. 320–52.

[26] Greene B. Ethnic minority lesbians and gay men: mental health and treatment issues. In: Greene B, editor. Ethnic and cultural diversity among lesbians and gay men. Thousand Oaks (CA): Sage; 1997. p. 216–39.

[27] Wilson PA, Yoshikawa H. Improving access to health care among African-American, Asian and Pacific Islander, and Latino LGB populations. In: Meyer IH, Northridge M, editors. The health of sexual minorities: public health perspectives on lesbian, gay, bisexual, and transgender populations. New York: Springer; 2007. p. 609–37.

[28] Eliason MJ, Shope R. Does "Don't Ask, Don't Tell" apply to health care? Lesbian, gay, and bisexual people's disclosure to health care providers. J Gay Lesbian Med Assoc 2001;5(4): 125–34.

[29] Lucas VA. An investigation of the health care preferences of the lesbian population. Health Care Women Int 1992;13(2):221–8.

[30] Barbara AM, Quandt SA, Anderson R. Experiences of lesbians in the health care environment. Women Health 2001;34(1):45–61.

[31] Meckler GD, Elliott MN, Kanouse DE, et al. Nondisclosure of sexual orientation to a physician among a sample of gay, lesbian, and bisexual youth. Arch Pediatr Adolesc Med 2006; 160(12):1248–54.

[32] Herek GM, Chopp R, Strohl D. Sexual stigma: putting sexual minority health issues in context. In: Meyer IH, Northridge M, editors. The health of sexual minorities: public health perspectives on lesbian, gay, bisexual, and transgender populations. New York: Springer; 2007. p. 151–208.

[33] Meyer IH. Prejudice, social stress, and mental health in lesbian, gay, and bisexual populations: conceptual issues and research evidence. Psychol Bull 2003;129(5):674–97.

[34] Szymanski D, Chung Y. Feminist attitudes and coping resources as correlates of lesbian internalized heterosexism. Fem Psychol 2003;13:369–89.

[35] Williamson IR. Internalized homophobia and health issues affecting lesbians and gay men. Health Educ Res 2000;15(1):97–107.

[36] Mays VM, Yancey AK, Cochran SD, et al. Heterogeneity of health disparities among African American, Hispanic, and Asian American women: unrecognized influences of sexual orientation. Am J Public Health 2002;92(4):632–9.

[37] Williams DR, Neighbors HW, Jackson JS. Racial/ethnic discrimination and health: findings from community studies. Am J Public Health 2003;93(2):200–8.

[38] Yoshikawa H, Wilson PA, Chae DH, et al. Do family and friendship networks protect against the influence of discrimination on mental health and HIV risk among Asian and Pacific Islander gay men? AIDS Educ Prev 2004;16(1):84–100.

[39] Díaz RM, Ayala G. Social discrimination and health outcomes: the case of Latino gay men and HIV risk. New York: National Gay and Lesbian Task Force, Policy Institute; 2001.

[40] Amadio DM. Internalized heterosexism, alcohol use, and alcohol-related problems among lesbians and gay men. Addict Behav 2006;31(7):1153–62.

[41] McKirnan DJ, Peterson PL. Alcohol and drug use among homosexual men and women: epidemiology and population characteristics. Addict Behav 1989;14(5):545–53.

[42] Hellman RE. Issues in the treatment of lesbian women and gay men with chronic mental illness. Psychiatr Serv 1996;47(10):1093–8.

[43] Coates T. Depression, gay men, and HIV acquisition. Focus 2004;19(10):5–6.

[44] Igartua KJ, Gill K, Montoro R. Internalized homophobia: a factor in depression, anxiety, and suicide in the gay and lesbian population. Can J Commun Ment Health 2003;22(2): 15–30.

[45] Koh AS, Ross LK. Mental health issues: a comparison of lesbian, bisexual and heterosexual women. J Homosex 2006;51(1):33–57.

[46] Hughes TL, Eliason MJ. Substance use and abuse in lesbian, gay, bisexual, and transgender populations. J Prim Prev 2002;22(3):261–95.

[47] Gruskin EP, Gordon N. Gay/lesbian sexual orientation increases risk for cigarette smoking and heavy drinking among members of a large Northern California health plan. BMC Public Health 2006;6:1–6. Available at: http://www.pubmedcentral.nih.gov/articlerender. fcgi?artid=1617098 or http://www.pubmedcentral.nih.gov/picrender.fcgi?artid=1617098& blobtype=pdf.

[48] Heck JE, Jacobson JS. Asthma diagnosis among individuals in same-sex relationships. J Asthma 2006;43(8):579–84.

[49] Maccio EM, Doueck H. Meeting the needs of the gay and lesbian community: outcomes in the human services. Journal of Gay and Lesbian Social Services 2002;14(4):55–73.

[50] Malebranche DJ, Peterson JL, Fullilove RE, et al. Race and sexual identity: perceptions about medical culture and healthcare among Black men who have sex with men. J Natl Med Assoc 2004;96(1):97–107.

[51] Stevens PE. The experiences of lesbians of color in health care encounters. J Lesbian Stud 1998;2(1):77–94.

[52] Kerker BD, Mostashari F, Thorpe L. Health care access and utilization among women who have sex with women: sexual behavior and identity. J Urban Health 2006;83(5):970–9.

[53] Matthews AK, Brandenburg DL, Johnson TP, et al. Correlates of underutilization of gyne-cological cancer screening among lesbian and heterosexual women. Prev Med 2004;38(1): 105–13.

[54] Bakker FC, Sandfort TG, Vanwesenbeeck I, et al. Do homosexual persons use health care services more frequently than heterosexual persons: findings from a Dutch population sur-vey. Soc Sci Med 2006;63(8):2022–30.

[55] Roberts SA, Dibble SL, Nussey B, et al. Cardiovascular disease risk in lesbian women. Womens Health Issues 2003;13(4):167–74.

[56] Ulstad V. Coronary health issues for lesbians. J Gay Lesbian Med Assoc 1999;3(2):59–66.

[57] Wang J, Hausermann M, Vounatsou P, et al. Health status, behavior, and care utilization in the Geneva Gay Men's Health Survey. Prev Med 2007;44(1):70–5.

[58] Case P, Austin SB, Hunter DJ, et al. Sexual orientation, health risk factors, and physical functioning in the Nurses' Health Study II. J Womens Health (Larchmt) 2004;13(9): 1033–47.

[59] Dibble SL, Roberts SA, Nussey B. Comparing breast cancer risk between lesbians and their heterosexual sisters. Womens Health Issues 2004;14(2):60–8.

[60] Aaron DJ, Markovic N, Danielson ME, et al. Behavioral risk factors for disease and preven-tive health practices among lesbians. Am J Public Health 2001;91(6):972–5.

[61] Engels EA. Infectious agents as causes of non-Hodgkin lymphoma. Cancer Epidemiol Bio-markers Prev 2007.

[62] Goldstone S. Anal dysplasia in men who have sex with men. AIDS Read 1999;9(3):204–8, 220.

[63] Martro E, Esteve A, Schulz TF, et al. Risk factors for human Herpesvirus 8 infection and AIDS-associated Kaposi's sarcoma among men who have sex with men in a European multi-centre study. Int J Cancer 2007;120(5):1129–35.

[64] CDC. HIV/AIDS among men who have sex with men. Available at: http://www.cdc.gov/hiv/topics/msm/resources/factsheets/msm.htm. Accessed March 13, 2007.

[65] Catalan J, Meadows J. Sexual dysfunction in gay and bisexual men with HIV infection: evaluation, treatment and implications. AIDS Care 2000;12(3):279–86.

[66] Rosen RC, Catania JA, Ehrhardt AA, et al. The Bolger conference on PDE-5 inhibition and HIV risk: implications for health policy and prevention. J Sex Med 2006;3(6):960–75, [discussion 973–965]. Available at: http://www.metlife.com/WPSAssets/15374435731164 722885V1FOutandAging.pdf.

[67] Blank TO. Gay men and prostate cancer: invisible diversity. J Clin Oncol 2005;23(12): 2593–6.

[68] Romanelli F, Smith KM. Recreational use of sildenafil by HIV-positive and -negative homosexual/bisexual males. Ann Pharmacother 2004;38(6):1024–30.

[69] Mansergh G, Shouse RL, Marks G, et al. Methamphetamine and sildenafil (Viagra) use are linked to unprotected receptive and insertive anal sex, respectively, in a sample of men who have sex with men. Sex Transm Infect 2006;82(2):131–4.

[70] Paul JP, Pollack L, Osmond D, et al. Viagra (sildenafil) use in a population-based sample of U.S. men who have sex with men. Sex Transm Dis 2005;32(9):531–3.

[71] Sanchez TH, Gallagher KM. Factors associated with recent sildenafil (Viagra) use among men who have sex with men in the United States. J Acquir Immune Defic Syndr 2006; 42(1):95–100.

[72] O'Toole CJ. The view from below: developing a knowledge base about an unknown popu-lation. Sex Disabil 2000;18(3):207–24.

[73] Eliason MJ. Substance abuse counsellor's attitudes regarding lesbian, gay, bisexual, and transgendered clients. J Subst Abuse 2000;12(4):311–28.

[74] Stevens PE, Hall JM. Stigma, health beliefs and experiences with health care in lesbian women. Image J Nurs Sch 1988;20(2):69–73.

[75] Geddes VA. Lesbian expectations and experiences with family doctors. How much does the physician's sex matter to lesbians? Can Fam Physician 1994;40:908–20.

[76] Röndahl G, Innala SM, Carlsson M. Heterosexual assumptions in verbal and non-verbal communication in nursing. J Adv Nurs 2006;56(4):373–81.

[77] Matthews AK, Hughes TL, Osterman GP, et al. Complementary medicine practices in a community-based sample of lesbian and heterosexual women. Health Care Women Int 2005;26(5):430–47.

[78] London AS, Foote-Ardah CE, Fleishman JA, et al. Use of alternative therapists among people in care for HIV in the United States. Am J Public Health 2003;93(6):980–7.

[79] Basson R, Schultz WW. Sexual sequelae of general medical disorders. Lancet 2007; 369(9559):409–24.

[80] Bitzer J, Platano G, Tschudin S, et al. Sexual counseling for women in the context of physical diseases: a teaching model for physicians. J Sex Med 2007;4(1):29–37.

[81] Reynolds KE, Magnan MA. Nursing attitudes and beliefs toward human sexuality: collaborative research promoting evidence-based practice. Clin Nurse Spec 2005;19(5):255–9.

[82] Magnan MA, Reynolds K. Barriers to addressing patient sexuality concerns across five areas of specialization. Clin Nurse Spec 2006;20(6):285–92.

[83] The MetLife Mature Market Institute®, in conjunction with the Lesbian and Gay Aging Issues Network of the American Society on Aging and Zogby International. Out and aging: the Metlife study of lesbian and gay baby boomers. Westport (CT): The MetLife Mature Market Institute®; 2006.

[84] Newman F. The whole lesbian sex book: a passionate guide for all of us. San Francisco (CA): Cleis Press; 2004.

[85] Silverstein C, Picano F. The joy of gay sex. 3rd edition. New York: Harper Collins Publishers; 2004.

ELSEVIER
SAUNDERS

NURSING
CLINICS
OF NORTH AMERICA

Nurs Clin N Am 42 (2007) 675–684

Sexuality and Spinal Cord Injury

Richard Ricciardi, PhD, NP, FAANP[a,b,*],
Christina M. Szabo, MS, CNRN, CCRN[c],
Amy Yribarren Poullos, BSN, RN[d]

[a]Walter Reed Army Medical Center, P.O. Box 59645, Walter Reed Station,
Washington, DC 20012, USA
[b]Uniformed Services University of the Health Sciences, 4301 Jones Bridge Road,
Bethesda, MD 20814, USA
[c]Virginia Commonwealth University Health System, 1250 East Marshall Street,
Richmond, VA 23294, USA
[d]San Carlos, CA, USA

The happiness of a [person] in this life does not consist in the absence but in
the mastery of [his or her] passions.

—Alfred Lord Tennyson

In the United States, more than 250,000 people are living with spinal cord
injury (SCI). Each year, approximately 10,000 new SCIs occur, with most individuals being between 16 and 30 years of age at the time of SCI presentation. SCI is most often the result of direct trauma to the spinal cord, but can
also be associated with congenital or degenerative disease [1]. As a result of
SCI, individuals experience physical and psychologic consequences that have
a profound impact on their sexual health. The impact on sexual functioning
depends on the degree of injury and its location on the spinal cord [2–4].

Both men and women report a significant decrease in sexual desire [4–6]
and frequency of sexual activity [7] after SCI. In men, the most common factors are erectile dysfunction and impaired ejaculation [8,9], and in women,
the most common factors are pain with intercourse and inability to reach
orgasm [10,11]. Erectile dysfunction is defined as the inability to achieve
or maintain an erection sufficient for satisfactory sexual activity [12].

Although patients and health care professionals have identified sexuality
and reproductive health as important aspects of SCI rehabilitation, gaps

The opinions and assertions contained herein are the private views of the authors and are
not to be construed as official or as reflecting the views of the Department of Defense or the
US Government.

* Corresponding author.
E-mail address: Richard.Ricciardi@us.army.mil (R. Ricciardi).

0029-6465/07/$ - see front matter. Published by Elsevier Inc.
doi:10.1016/j.cnur.2007.08.005
nursing.theclinics.com

exist in knowledge, in the clinical skills necessary for the assessment of a patient's sexual health, and in providing education on sexual health during the rehabilitation process [13,14]. As part of the rehabilitation health care team, nurses are in a strong position to address the sexuality and reproductive health needs of the SCI patient and to conduct research to provide an evidence-based approach to short- and long-term care.

Physiologic changes in the spinal cord–injured patient

The effects on sexual physiology depend on the type, level, and degree of the SCI and whether the damage to the sacral spinal segments is an upper or lower motor neuron injury. In general, an intact neural system is required for a successful and complete erection. Penile erection occurs by two mechanisms: reflex erection caused by direct touching of the penile shaft, and psychogenic erection, which occurs by erotic stimuli [15]. Reflex erection involves the peripheral nerves and the lower parts of the spinal cord, whereas psychogenic erection involves the limbic system of the brain.

Male sexual functioning after SCI impairments centers on erection, ejaculation, and fertility. Most men with SCI experience impairments in psychogenic erections. Men with complete upper motor neuron lesions may have reflex erections in response to physical contact, but no psychogenic erection. Men with an incomplete upper motor neuron injury maintain the ability to have reflex erections and may also experience psychogenic erections, although they may not be sufficient for intercourse [16]. Approximately 25% of men with complete lower motor neuron lesions of the sacral spinal segment may have psychogenic erections and may be able to ejaculate; however, reflex erections are unlikely [17].

Several options exist for the treatment of erectile dysfunction in patients who have SCI. Oral phosphodiesterase-5 inhibitors (PDE-5 inhibitors) such as sildenafil, vardenafil, and tadalafil are effective and well tolerated in the SCI population. These drugs enhance the quality and duration of erection and may increase the frequency of reflex and psychogenic erections [18,19]. In cases where oral therapy is ineffective, intracavernous injections of vasoactive substances such as papaverine, alone or in combination with phentolamine or prostaglandin E 1 [20,21], may be used [3,9]. Alternatively, vacuum pumps can produce an erection and, when used in conjunction with constriction rings that occlude venous outflow, the erection is sustained [22]. With the advent of oral pharmacologic agents for the treatment of erectile dysfunction, male SCI patients infrequently resort to penile implants. Penile prostheses continue to be used for complex penile reconstruction and for erectile dysfunction that does not respond to oral pharmacologic therapy or pharmacologic agents injected into the corpus cavernosum [23].

In addition to having problems with erectile dysfunction, ejaculatory function may be compromised in SCI because of an impairment in the coordinated neurologic impulses between the sympathetic, parasympathetic, and somatic nervous systems [24,25]. Ejaculation and orgasm are likely to occur simultaneously, although a number of men with SCI achieve orgasm without ejaculation [26]. Men with incomplete SCI are more likely to achieve simultaneous orgasm and ejaculation than those with complete SCI. Men with complete lower motor neuron dysfunction affecting their sacral segments are less likely to achieve orgasm than men with any other patterns of SCI [25,27].

Male infertility associated with SCI occurs from a combination of erectile dysfunction and ejaculatory failure. In the acute phase of SCI, semen quality is normal (6–12 days postinjury) but over time, sperm motility and viability declines [28]. Nurses should provide counseling to the male SCI patient and his family that using electro-ejaculation (induction of ejaculation by gradually increasing electric current delivered through a probe inserted into the rectum) during the acute phase of SCI can provide normal serum for banking [28,29]. Once sperm is banked, it can be used for in vitro fertilization/intra-cytoplasmic sperm injection. Additional factors that contribute to infertility include frequent urinary tract infections, impaired scrotal thermoregulation, medications, retrograde ejaculation, and changes in seminal fluid [17,30].

In general, female sexuality after SCI has received far less attention and research than male sexual issues. In women with SCI, sexual function centers on the impairments in the pathways of female sexual arousal, which are manifested by changes in vaginal vasocongestion, vasoconstriction, and lubrication [10]. Women with complete upper motor neuron injury experience reflexic vaginal vasocongestion but not psychogenic vaginal vasocongestion. They do, however, experience increased vaginal vasoconstriction and lubrication with tactile stimulation. Women with incomplete upper motor neuron injuries experience reflexic and psychogenic vaginal lubrication. Women with complete lower motor neuron injuries report psychogenic lubrication but not reflex lubrication. Women with incomplete lower motor neuron injuries may have both psychogenic and reflex vaginal lubrication [17,31]. In addition, after SCI, women report that they have difficulty becoming psychologically and physically sexually aroused and that their SCI altered their sexual sense of self [32].

In contrast to an abundant research into fertility in male SCI patients, research into fertility in women with SCI is sparse. Some case reports and expert opinion indicate that female fertility is primarily unaffected by SCI. More research is needed in this area. Amenorrhea is reported in 50% to 60% of all women in the acute phase of SCI; however, within 6 months of injury, approximately 50%, and after 1 year, approximately 90%, of women have resumed their normal menstrual cycle [17]. It is presumed that once an SCI woman has resumed menses, pregnancy is possible. When addressing birth control options in SCI women, consideration must be given to the physical limitations and physiologic consequences of the SCI. Oral contraceptives may be contraindicated because of the potential increased risk of venous thrombosis [33].

After SCI, some women may believe that they become infertile or that they can no longer give birth to a healthy child. These misconceptions should be corrected by intervening early with reproductive education. No matter what the level or severity of spinal cord impairment, women with SCI frequently do have healthy children [34,35]. However, true pregnancy rates and frequency of miscarriages are unknown because of the lack of prior or ongoing research.

In addition to the gender-specific changes in the SCI patient, physical changes impact women and men and their ability and willingness to participate in sexual activity [36,37]. Bladder function, which depends on an intact autonomic nervous system, is altered in SCI. Urine leakage or "accidents" are possible during all stages of sexual arousal and activity. Urinary odor and external drainage devices may negatively impact desire, libido, and sexual arousal. SCI patients may experience bowel incontinence and flatulence during sexual activity. The possibility of autonomic dysreflexia affecting bladder and bowel function, cardiovascular control, and temperature regulation may diminish willingness to engage in sexual activity. Because of alterations in thermoregulation, the SCI patient may be physically uncomfortable being unclothed. In addition, the appearance and texture of the skin and the risk for skin breakdown not only limit sexual positioning but greatly affect comfort with body image [18].

Patients who have SCI experience a loss of muscle tone, which, in addition to affecting body image, limits the ability to touch, cuddle, and hold a partner. Further, the reduced capability to balance and support the body imposes limits on sexual positioning and movement of the pelvis during intercourse. In addition, sudden muscle spasms can interrupt sexual activity and restrict positioning. Further, neuropathic pain may inhibit participation and enjoyment of sexual activity [18,38,39].

Adaptation to spinal cord injury

Healthy sexual adjustment following SCI requires adaptation to a changed physical body. SCI patients must redefine their ideas about who they are as sexual beings (ie, their sexual self-concepts). Individuals and society have established views of what is normal and acceptable sexual behavior. The dominant view is that sexuality is a privilege of the able-bodied. Disabled individuals are often treated by society like children in need of protection and, therefore, unlikely candidates for sexual expression and reproduction. These social and cultural attitudes can be as disabling as the physical limitations of SCI [40]. Table 1 provides an overview of problems associated with SCI and suggested nursing interventions.

Much of the early research conduced on sexuality in the SCI patient has been performed on men, focusing on physiologic changes and medical treatments. Recent literature has provided insight into the psychologic impact of

SCI, specifically evaluating sexual satisfaction and predictors of positive outcomes [4,18,32]. In a prospective, longitudinal study of sexual health among people with spinal cord injuries, Fisher and colleagues [41] administered questionnaires to 32 men and eight women at four intervals between initial inpatient rehabilitation and 18 months postdischarge. Researchers found that 17 of the participants resumed sexual activity within 6 months of injury and 23 were sexually active at 12 months. Sexual adjustment was found to improve over time, and fewer sexual concerns were reported. Low levels of sexual desire and arousal were reported by approximately one half of the participants, but only one third reported sexual dissatisfaction. Participant concerns about sexuality focused on performance issues, the ability to attract a partner, feeling or inflicting physical or emotional pain, and managing the practical issues of when and where to engage in sexual activity. Although few participants sought sexual counseling beyond that offered during rehabilitation, identified educational needs included coping with changes in sexual functioning, methods and techniques to achieve sexual satisfaction and improve function, partner support, and attitudes toward sexuality. Satisfaction with sexual activity and the level of intimacy, quantity, and type of social interactions were positively correlated. In other words, higher social integration was associated with higher sexual satisfaction.

Other studies support the importance of relationships and sexual satisfaction among SCI patients. In a study of sexual adjustment and quality of relationships in SCI patients, a team of researchers administered questionnaires to 64 men and 11 women with SCI [6]. The 80-item instrument assessed dimensions of sexuality and aspects of the emotional quality of relationships. Researchers found that, although SCI patients reported lower sexual activity and satisfaction compared with healthy controls, the quality of relationships was similar. In both the SCI and control groups, having a diverse repertoire of sexual expression, and sexual satisfaction, were positively correlated. In both groups, perceived partner satisfaction and sexual satisfaction were also positively correlated. The ability and willingness to adapt to new ways of sexual expression were particularly important among SCI patients. Continued, but decreased, sexual activity was reported among the SCI participants, citing physical limitations as the main barrier. Participants in the control group also reported decreased sexual activity, citing relationship problems, fatigue, and lack of time as the main barriers, suggesting that sexuality is affected by many factors besides disability.

Nursing intervention includes fostering two-way and open communication on sexual intimacy issues between SCI patients and their partners. Identifying new erogenous zones and sexual positions by exploration and communication between partners is critical to returning to a fulfilling sexual life after SCI. Patients will most likely not be able use all of the coital positions that were used before SCI. It is only through personal exploration and communication that new coital positions will be identified. In SCI women,

Table 1
Problems associated with spinal cord injury and nursing interventions

Problem area	Cause	Nursing interventions
Erection	Complete and incomplete upper or lower motor neuron injury causing changes in reflex and psychogenic erections	Inform patients of pharmacologic options: oral PDE-5 inhibitors (sildenafil, vardenafil, tadalafil), intracavernous injections of vasoactive substances; provide information on vacuum pumps, constriction rings, and penile implants; encourage discussion about methods of enhancing sexual arousal/psychogenic erections.
Ejaculation	Impairment of coordinated neurologic impulses among sympathetic, parasympathetic, and somatic nervous systems	Provide information on electro-ejaculation procedure.
Male fertility	Erectile dysfunction; ejaculatory failure; frequent urinary tract infections; impaired scrotal thermoregulation; medications; retrograde ejaculation; changes in seminal fluid	Discuss cryopreservation through electro-ejaculation in acute phase; discuss intrauterine insemination, in vitro fertilization, and in vitro fertilization with intracytoplasmic sperm injection.
Female sexual arousal	Complete and incomplete upper or lower motor neuron injury, causing changes in reflexic and psychogenic vaginal vasoconstriction, vasocongestion, and lubrication	Address benefits of tactile stimulation; provide education and discussion about methods of enhancing sexual arousal.
Female fertility	Unaffected by SCI? (research is sparse)	Discuss and debunk misconceptions; provide reproductive education to address physical limitations and physiologic implications of pregnancy; discuss birth control options and potential contraindications of oral contraceptives (increased risk of venous thrombosis).
Sexual self-concept	Changes in physical appearance; limited sexual positioning; autonomic dysreflexia; urinary and bowel incontinence; decreased thermoregulation; spasticity; pain	Encourage creativity regarding sexual positions; encourage use of "toys"; provide information on medication for pain and spasticity; introduce bowel training schedule and intermittent catheterization schedule to control incontinence; encourage communication and partner support; facilitate referral of patients to counseling.
Pediatric/adolescent sexual development	Societal barriers; functional limitations	Provide developmentally appropriate sexual education; involve family and social networks in plan of care.

having the partner on top during coitus may work well; however, caution must be used so as not to put too much weight on the chest, which could incite breathing difficulties. Some women like this position best because there is direct clitoral stimulation. In SCI men, coital positions such as sitting in a chair that has arms for support or in a wheelchair may work well. Lying down on the side or back may also work well. Some SCI patients may feel lying on their side or back provides additional energy for coitus because less energy is used to support their weight. Further, lying on the side or back also provides free hands to help with stimulation.

If the SCI patient has a urinary catheter, it is best to empty the bladder and remove the catheter before coitus. If the urinary catheter cannot be removed because of medical reasons, then, in women, the catheter may be taped to the stomach. In SCI men, the catheter tube can be folded and taped over the penis or held in place by a condom on an erect penis.

Spinal cord injury and the pediatric/adolescent patient

The epidemiologic characteristics of SCI in the pediatric population are distinctly different from the adult population. Using data collected from the Kids' Inpatient Database developed as part of the Healthcare Cost and Utilization Project sponsored by the Agency for Healthcare Research and Quality and the National Trauma Database, significant differences in the annual incidence rate of pediatric and adolescent SCI were found to exist between patient populations stratified by race and sex. The rate of SCI in African Americans was 1.53 cases per 100,000; in Native Americans, 1.0 case per 100,000; in Hispanics, 0.87 case per 100,000; and in Asians, 0.36 case per 100,000. Also, the incidence in boys is more than twice as high as in girls. Frequency of SCI remained constant until 12 years of age, at which point it rose steeply until 18 years of age. Overall, the incidence of pediatric and adolescent SCI in the United States is 1.99 cases per 100,000. From these data, 1455 pediatric and adolescent patients are estimated to be admitted to American hospitals each year for treatment of SCI [42,43].

As mentioned previously, the predominance of research on SCI and sexuality has been conducted on men, leaving many gaps in providing evidence-based care to pediatric and adolescent patients who have SCI. Regardless of the age at which a child sustains SCI, the challenge for parents, nurses, and the health care and educational team is in providing opportunities for the pediatric and adolescent SCI patient to development normally, along with his/her peers. In a review of sexuality in children with disabilities [44], adolescents with disabilities frequently participate in sexual relationships without the adequate knowledge and skills to keep them healthy, safe, and satisfied. Although sexual development in physically disabled pediatric and adolescent patients may be hindered by functional limitations and societal barriers, opportunities to develop into sexually expressive and fulfilled persons can and do exist. To serve SCI pediatric and adolescent patients best, parents, family, and the educational and health care team need to take a proactive approach in implementing evidence-based strategies that promote the physical, emotional, social, and psychosexual independence of children and adolescents with SCI. In addition, nurses are well positioned to refer families and patients to pediatric and adolescent SCI centers that offer sexuality education as part of a comprehensive rehabilitation program.

Summary

The impact of SCI on sexuality depends greatly on the degree of injury and the location of the injury on the spinal cord. Sexual dysfunction has physiologic and psychologic causes and its effect is influenced by the patient's age, gender, culture, and comorbid medical conditions. Although sexual satisfaction, desire, and frequency of intercourse decline in sexually active patients after SCI, a positive adjustment has been reported by most SCI patients over time. Sexual satisfaction and fulfillment are greater in patients who are engaged in a strong emotional relationship with good communication and who are open to sexual experimentation, and when the patient perceives that his/her partner enjoys the sexual aspects of their relationship.

In the pediatric and adolescent SCI patient, developmentally appropriate sexuality education should be initiated early in the rehabilitation process. In addition, strengthening skills in communication, decision-making, and understanding normal sexual health and development are integral to the sexual rehabilitation and relationship process. A team approach among health care and educational professionals, parents or guardians, faith-based groups, and the patient and his/her peer group assists in promoting normal development in an environment that fosters safe and healthy sexual practices. The ultimate goal of the rehabilitation process is for children to develop into socially and sexually well adjusted adults.

Using a holistic developmental team approach to care, the nurse is well positioned to address the acute and long-term rehabilitation needs of the SCI patient. By assisting SCI patients through the grieving process and promoting a positive, yet realistic, self-concept, nurses can mitigate potential problems in body image disturbances, decreased self-esteem, and gender-specific sexuality issues.

References

[1] Ho CH, Wuermser LA, Priebe MM, et al. Spinal cord injury medicine. 1. Epidemiology and classification. Arch Phys Med Rehabil 2007;88(3 Suppl 1):S49–54.
[2] Dikaios S. If not the disability, then what? Barriers to reclaiming sexuality following spinal cord injury. Sex Disabil 2006;24(2):101–11.

[3] Deforge D, Blackmer J, Garritty C, et al. Male erectile dysfunction following spinal cord injury: a systematic review. Spinal Cord 2006;44(8):465–73.

[4] Forsythe E, Horsewell JE. Sexual rehabilitation of women with a spinal cord injury. Spinal Cord 2006;44(4):234–41.

[5] Reitz A, Tobe V, Knapp PA, et al. Impact of spinal cord injury on sexual health and quality of life. Int J Impot Res 2004;16(2):167–74.

[6] Kreuter M, Sullivan M, Siosteen A. Sexual adjustment and quality of relationship in spinal paraplegia: a controlled study. Arch Phys Med Rehabil 1996;77(6):541–8.

[7] Sipski ML, Alexander CJ. Sexual activities, response and satisfaction in women pre- and post-spinal cord injury. Arch Phys Med Rehabil 1993;74(10):1025–9.

[8] Ramos AS, Samso JV. Specific aspects of erectile dysfunction in spinal cord injury. Int J Impot Res 2004;16(Suppl 2):S42–5.

[9] Monga M, Bernie J, Rajasekaran M. Male infertility and erectile dysfunction in spinal cord injury: a review. Arch Phys Med Rehabil 1999;80(10):1331–9.

[10] Sipski ML, Alexander CJ, Rosen R. Sexual arousal and orgasm in women: effects of spinal cord injury. Ann Neurol 2001;49(1):35–44.

[11] Ferreiro-Velasco ME, Barca-Buyo A, de la Barrera SS, et al. Sexual issues in a sample of women with spinal cord injury. Spinal Cord 2005;43(1):51–5.

[12] Smith EM, Bodner DR. Sexual dysfunction after spinal cord injury. Urol Clin North Am 1993;20(3):535–42.

[13] McAlonan S. Improving sexual rehabilitation services: the patient's perspective. Am J Occup Ther 1996;50(10):826–34.

[14] Kroll T, Beatty PW, Bingham S. Primary care satisfaction among adults with physical disabilities: the role of patient-provider communication. Manag Care Q 2003;11(1):11–9.

[15] Ramos AS, Samso JV. Specific aspects of erectile dysfunction in spinal cord injury. Int J Impot Res 2004;16(Suppl 2):S42–5.

[16] Biering-Sorensen F, Sonksen J. Sexual function in spinal cord lesioned men. Spinal Cord 2001;39(9):455–70.

[17] Linsenmeyer TA. Sexual function and infertility following spinal cord injury. Phys Med Rehabil Clin N Am 2000;11(1):141–56, ix.

[18] Elliott SL. Problems of sexual function after spinal cord injury. Prog Brain Res 2006;152: 387–99.

[19] Derry F, Hultling C, Seftel AD, et al. Efficacy and safety of sildenafil citrate (Viagra) in men with erectile dysfunction and spinal cord injury: a review. Urology 2002;60(2 Suppl 2):49–57.

[20] Meinhardt W, de la Fuente RB, Lycklama a Nijeholt AA, et al. Prostaglandin E1 with phentolamine for the treatment of erectile dysfunction. Int J Impot Res 1996;8(1):5–7.

[21] Shamloul R, Atteya A, Elnashaar A, et al. Intracavernous sodium nitroprusside (SNP) versus papaverine/phentolamine in erectile dysfunction: a comparative study of short-term efficacy and side-effects. J Sex Med 2005;2(1):117–20.

[22] Lewis RW, Witherington R. External vacuum therapy for erectile dysfunction: use and results. World J Urol 1997;15(1):78–82.

[23] Carson CC. Penile prosthesis implantation: surgical implants in the era of oral medication. Urol Clin North Am 2005;32(4):503–9, vii.

[24] Sipski ML. Sexual functioning in the spinal cord injured. Int J Impot Res 1998;10(Suppl 2): S128–30, [discussion: S138–40].

[25] Johnson RD. Descending pathways modulating the spinal circuitry for ejaculation: effects of chronic spinal cord injury. Prog Brain Res 2006;152:415–26.

[26] Sipski M, Alexander CJ, Gomez-Marin O. Effects of level and degree of spinal cord injury on male orgasm. Spinal Cord 2006;44(12):798–804.

[27] Allard J, Truitt WA, McKenna KE, et al. Spinal cord control of ejaculation. World J Urol 2005;23(2):119–26.

[28] Brown DJ, Hill ST, Baker HW. Male fertility and sexual function after spinal cord injury. Prog Brain Res 2006;152:427–39.

[29] Das S, Soni BM, Sharma SD, et al. A case of rapid deterioration in sperm quality following spinal cord injury. Spinal Cord 2006;44(1):56–8.

[30] Linsenmeyer TA, Perkash I. Infertility in men with spinal cord injury. Arch Phys Med Rehabil 1991;72(10):747–54.

[31] Sipski ML, Arenas A. Female sexual function after spinal cord injury. Prog Brain Res 2006; 152:441–7.

[32] Anderson KD, Borisoff JF, Johnson RD, et al. Spinal cord injury influences psychogenic as well as physical components of female sexual ability. Spinal Cord 2007;45(5):349–59.

[33] Anderson FA Jr, Spencer FA. Risk factors for venous thromboembolism. Circulation 2003; 107(23 Suppl 1):I9–16.

[34] Jackson AB, Lindsey LL, Klebine PL, et al. Reproductive health for women with spinal cord injury: pregnancy and delivery. SCI Nurs 2004;21(2):88–91.

[35] Deforge D, Blackmer J, Moher D, et al. Sexuality and reproductive health following spinal cord injury. Evid Rep Technol Assess (Summ) 2004;109(109):1–8.

[36] Black K, Sipski ML, Strauss SS. Sexual satisfaction and sexual drive in spinal cord injured women. J Spinal Cord Med 1998;21(3):240–4.

[37] Phelps G, Brown M, Chen J, et al. Sexual experience and plasma testosterone levels in male veterans after spinal cord injury. Arch Phys Med Rehabil 1983;64(2):47–52.

[38] Valtonen K, Karlsson AK, Siosteen A, et al. Satisfaction with sexual life among persons with traumatic spinal cord injury and meningomyelocele. Disabil Rehabil 2006;28(16):965–76.

[39] Anderson KD, Borisoff JF, Johnson RD, et al. The impact of spinal cord injury on sexual function: concerns of the general population. Spinal Cord 2007;45(5):328–37.

[40] Mitchell ST. Sexuality and disability: the missing discourse of pleasure. Sex Disabil 2000; 18(4):283–90.

[41] Fisher TL, Laud PW, Byfield MG, et al. Sexual health after spinal cord injury: a longitudinal study. Arch Phys Med Rehabil 2002;83(8):1043–51.

[42] DeVivo MJ, Vogel LC. Epidemiology of spinal cord injury in children and adolescents. J Spinal Cord Med 2004;27(Suppl 1):S4–10.

[43] Burke DA, Linden RD, Zhang YP, et al. Incidence rates and populations at risk for spinal cord injury: a regional study. Spinal Cord 2001;39(5):274–8.

[44] Murphy N. Sexuality in children and adolescents with disabilities. Dev Med Child Neurol 2005;47(9):640–4.

NURSING
CLINICS
OF NORTH AMERICA

ELSEVIER
SAUNDERS

Nurs Clin N Am 42 (2007) 685–696

Including Sexuality in Your Nursing Practice

Judith A. Shell, PhD, LMFT, RN

Osceola Cancer Center, 737 West Oak Street, Kissimmee, FL 34741, USA

Sexuality is a topic of great interest today, given the exposure in the electronic and print media, and one would think that this exposure would elevate the medical professional's comfort level with communication regarding sexuality issues. However, writers continue to comment on clinician discomfort or lack of discussion with their patients about sexual concerns and anxieties [1,2]. And, perhaps because of the media in general, if a discussion around sexuality does occur, it is often reserved for the young and healthy because the needs of people in their elder years, or those who face chronic physical illness or other functional alterations, are downplayed or felt to be less important.

Within the realm of cancer care, as one example of a chronic illness, if sexuality is discussed, this discussion is more likely to take place with those patients whose sexual function may be directly impacted (eg, cancer of the breast, cervix, prostate, testes, or colon). Patients who have other cancers, such as lung, gastric, or head and neck, may not be afforded communication about how these cancers may influence their sexuality and self-image [2,3]. Others who may be left out of a sexuality discussion are the elderly or gay, lesbian, bisexual, and transgendered individuals; even those of a different culture such as Hispanics, Asian Americans, Indian Americans, or those of European heritage may cause increased anxiety for the clinician. Nurses who care for chronically ill patients may help foster a more positive self-esteem for the patient, and may influence patient–partner attitudes about worthiness, self-concept, and body image, by providing opportunities to talk about feelings and fears about how treatment may affect their sexuality [3].

Even though their desire for survival may overshadow sexuality and a desire for intimacy immediately after a diagnosis of diseases such as diabetes, heart

---

E-mail address: shelljashell@aol.com

0029-6465/07/$ - see front matter © 2007 Elsevier Inc. All rights reserved.
doi:10.1016/j.cnur.2007.08.007
nursing.theclinics.com

disease, or cancer, many patients want to learn about the implications of their treatment and medications on their sexuality [4]. Patients are usually pursuing validation of their concerns and want to hear that other people have similar issues with intimacy and sexuality. They want practical advice so they can take control of their health and reaffirm themselves as sexual beings, and they want this advice from a health care professional whom they know, rather than by being referred to someone else [5,6]. Many times, patients are ignorant of some aspects of their sexuality and the nurse is in a position to enlighten them with valuable information. One study examined the questions men with prostate cancer wanted answered. From a possible list of 93 questions formulated by the researchers, 5 related to sexuality and included such matters as how treatment would affect sexual functioning and for how long, whether the cancer would worsen if the patient had sex, and whether the patient could have sex during treatment [7]. In an assessment of 73 women with gynecologic cancer, it was learned that 60% wanted more information, and more than 50% had received little or no information regarding how their sexuality might be affected by the cancer. These women (60.3%) preferred a personal discussion with their health care provider [8].

If the patient has a partner, communication with the couple together is important to treatment outcomes and relief of sexual distress. Changes in body image or self-perception can affect intimacy and social relationships, especially if there is a crisis during the illness [9]. The nurse plays a key role in encouraging patients to explore these changes in sexuality and intimacy with their partners. Providing assessment and guidance relating to the different types of treatment, resumption of sexual activity, and feelings of femininity and masculinity is imperative because most patients will not initiate this discussion. Kneece [10] reports that only about one third of 126 women who had surgery and chemotherapy for breast cancer asked their health care providers about sexual side effects, and the responses received were rated as insufficient. Professionals can no longer forget or avoid these discussions.

Attitudes and comfort levels of health care professionals

Sexuality is not a static concept and varies across time and place. Our ideas about normal and appropriate sexual behavior, whether these relate to gender roles, sexual identity, or the experience and expression of sexual desires, originate from the interaction of social and cultural forces [11]. Although the nurse may recognize the role of social factors in the sexual issues of their patients, they may fail to see their own cultural biases. Along with these biases comes the simple discomfort of talking about the patient's sexuality. Nurses rarely have difficulty talking about bowel habits, the most unpleasant side effects of treatment, or impending death, but they often stop short of discussing topics of a sexual nature, which may impair provision of total disease management. Often the attitude is, "It isn't my job," "It's too personal," "I never learned this in school," or "I might offend my patient" [4].

In an attempt to be at ease with a conversation regarding sexuality, the nurse may wish to explore several avenues, such as bibliotherapy; consultation with other nurses who are comfortable with sexuality; observation of those who incorporate sexual assessment into their practices; role-playing; attendance at seminars or workshops designed to assist in examination of attitudes, values, and beliefs about sexuality; or participating in a self-assessment for the professional (Box. 1) [4,12]. The development of good communication skills though role-playing, by asking questions that proceed from less sensitive to more sensitive issues is most helpful. It is suggested that the nurse take a set of questions and experiment with a friend, colleague, partner, or even a patient with whom he/she an established relationship. After several practice conversations with known and trusted people, comfort levels are often enhanced, and it becomes easier to ask questions or carry on a discussion about sexual issues.

Knowledge and education of the professional

Because most physicians and nurses have not had any type of sexuality training in school, an increase in one's sexual health knowledge is important. This knowledge may include studying textbooks and dedicated journals that deal with the topics of sexual anatomy and physiology, psychosexual development, the sexual response cycle, effects of aging on sexual functioning, and cultural, religious, and ethical implications [13]. In addition, a grasp of the range of human sexual expressions and behaviors assists the nurse in maintaining a nonjudgmental approach when caring for patients who practice nontraditional sexual behaviors [14]. Another method to enhance knowledge could be communication with other professionals in book and journal clubs. This method allows for interaction and the sharing of experiences and knowledge, along with other possible patient concerns that impact sexuality related to many chronic conditions, such as diabetes, hypertension, cancer, heart disease, and the medications used to control them [4].

Assessment: how and when

Ideally, a sexual assessment would be an in-depth, fact-finding mission that understands the context of the patient's life (ie, age, relationship status, living arrangement, career status, parental status, and much more) and would comprise questions about past and present sexual functioning, and intrapsychic, environmental, and interpersonal risk factors for sexual difficulty. These risk factors may include people who do not have a committed

---

Box 1. A guide to self-assessment for professionals

Level of comfort
Desensitization is used to increase the level of comfort. This
    process involves exposure to anxiety-producing material while
    in a relaxed atmosphere. It might include discussions about
    sexuality with trusted colleagues or attending a sexual attitude
    reassessment seminar. This process allows the professional to
    become more comfortable with dealing with sexuality.
    1. How comfortable do you feel discussing sexual matters?
    2. Notice physical tension, body position, eye contact, and
       facial expression when listening to specific sexual content.
       What content makes you feel uneasy?
    3. What sexual terms can you comfortably use to describe
       sexual fantasies, interest, arousal, orgasm, and behaviors?
       Try describing these experiences to a colleague.

Attitudes
The importance of knowing your sexual attitudes is to assess
    your ability to guide clients/patients regarding sexuality.
    Positive attitudes toward sexuality are important to
    communicate to patients.
    1. List three values you have about sexual behavior.
    2. How would these values affect the way you would work with
       clients/patients whose problems reflect a conflict with your
       values?
    3. List any areas regarding sexuality which are unacceptable to
       you.
    4. What could you do to compensate for your attitudes if
       a patient presented something in one of these areas?

Knowledge
A knowledge base about normal sexual functioning and the
    possible changes with cancer is important for assisting
    patients.

---

partner, those in already unhappy relationships, those who are younger and
will wish to have more children, and people who already have sexual problems or a history of sexual trauma like rape or molestation. However, most
nurses do not take this type of history, nor do they have the time to do so
[15]. Two particular models may be helpful and provide a guide to procure
and provide sexuality information for patients and partners. One model is
the PLISSIT model (P = permission, LI = limited information, SS = specific
suggestions, IT = intensive therapy), and the other is the BETTER model

(B = bring up the topic, E = explaining sexuality as part of quality of life, T = tell patient about appropriate resources, T = timing, E = educate about side effects, R = record in patient chart) (Table 1) [16,17]. Both models promote communication in a uniform manner, which usually increases confidence in the nurse and validates the patient. However, even these models may be seen as too cumbersome. Spaulding [18] explains that she uses one simple question during an initial assessment, which is, "Do you feel that your sexuality has changed since your diagnosis?" She further says that

Table 1
Sample sexual assessment questions and statements

PLISSIT model	BETTER model
Permission: Many patients who have heart disease have questions about how their treatment will affect their sexuality. Would you like to discuss that at this time?	*Bring up the topic:* Many patients who have diabetes have questions about how their treatment will affect their sexuality. What questions do you have at this time?
Limited information: Many women who take tamoxifen for breast cancer complain of a vaginal discharge or a dry vagina during intercourse. If you have problems with dryness, you may use a vaginal lubricant like Astroglide.	*Explain:* I am also concerned with sexuality, which is a quality-of-life issue like sleep or emotional contentment. I will answer your questions to the best of my ability.
Specific suggestions: Men who have had colorectal surgery like yours find they may get an erection and ejaculate, but have no discharge of semen. This situation is normal, and if you want to try to have children, specific techniques are available to obtain your sperm from your urine for artificial insemination or in vitro fertilization.	*Tell:* I understand you have several question about how your chemotherapy treatment will affect your ability to have children. I will obtain literature for you from Fertile Hope, which is a foundation that assists all cancer patients during and after treatment is finished with information and other resources.
Intensive therapy: Most nurses are not educated well enough to provide a patient and his/her partner with appropriate sex therapy. It is appropriate to refer these patients to a local therapist who is certified by the American Association of Sex Educators, Counselors, Therapists (AASECT) or who has experience with cancer patients regarding sexuality issues.	*Timing:* If the timing does not seem right during your first encounter with the patient, explain to him/her that you are willing to talk about sexuality issues and questions at any time during the treatment trajectory.
—	*Educate:* Give patients written materials along with verbal explanations regarding how their treatment will affect their sexual function. An excellent source for cancer patients is the American Cancer Society sexuality booklets written by Leslie Schover for men and women with cancer [40].
—	*Record:* Document all conversations, who was present (patient only or patient and partner), and educational materials given.

she informs her patient that she asks this question to all of her patients and she wants to increase his/her comfort in discussing these matters with her at any time, even if he/she does not want to talk about them during the present assessment. If an open-ended question is preferable, one can modify this question by asking, "What has your physician told you about how your heart attack will affect your sexuality?" or "What questions can I answer for you about how your medication will affect your sexuality?" An example of a specific, disease-related sexual assessment form is the International Index of Erectile Function, which ascertains pre-and posttreatment erectile function for prostate cancer patients [19]. Regardless of when assessment takes place or with what method, the guidelines in Table 2 will enhance patient and nurse comfort levels. Other strategies involve the timing of the assessment and counseling, use of predetermined interview questions, and phrasing responses in nonthreatening language.

Nine participants in a focus group conducted by Bruner and Boyd [20] of women treated for gynecologic or breast cancer commented on the timing of

Table 2
Sexuality assessment guidelines

Essential elements	How accomplished
Ensure privacy.	For in-patients, close the door or draw the curtain and speak in low tones, or move to another area, such as an office or conference room.
Ensure confidentiality.	Reassure the patient and partner that the conversation is confidential. Meet privately with the patient first unless otherwise requested, and then include the partner.
Address sexual concerns early and throughout treatment.	Initiate discussion early in the relationship, thereby implying that sexuality is an important component of good health. Use sexual terms before expecting the patient to use them. Use the patient's language.
Determine patient goals.	Remember that all patients do not experience sexual satisfaction in the same manner. A patient may not have a partner, or want one. Sexuality may not be a part of his/her concept of quality of life.
Avoid overreaction.	Listen to the patient with genuine interest, which conveys acceptance. Present a positive, relaxed attitude. Do not reveal shock or surprise with facial expressions. Keep personal feelings to yourself.
Refer patients for complex problems.	Know your referral sources and use them if a complex problem arises that is beyond the scope of help you can provide.

Adapted from Shell J. Impact of cancer on sexuality. In: Otto S, editor. Oncology nursing. 4th edition. St. Louis (MO): Mosby-Year Book, Inc.; 2001, p. 854.

a sexual assessment. Married women said that they would prefer to talk about sexuality issues after their treatment was finished (between 6 months and 1 year) because if they had received a questionnaire right after diagnosis, they would probably have thrown it away, whereas the two single women said they would have embraced the questionnaire immediately (one woman was in a relationship that was primarily sexual and it was an important aspect in her life). A study of 73 women with gynecologic cancer reported that 23.3% preferred information after diagnosis but before treatment, and 39.5% wanted information given after completion of treatment [8]. Mallinger and colleagues [21] agreed with these findings and also agreed that, during diagnosis and treatment, comprehension of medical information may be lacking and patients may be unable to verbalize their needs. These researchers advocate discussion of sexuality at various points along the treatment trajectory, rather than at one particular point in time. Also, a study of heterosexual couples by Sanders and colleagues [22] revealed that men think and respond differently from women to intimacy and relationship challenges that happen during treatment for prostate cancer. Consequently, the investigators recommended that health care providers working with prostate survivors must consider the unique relationship and intimacy needs for men and women. However, as Wilmoth [4] so aptly expressed, "One important caveat to talking about sexuality with your patients is that most of the conversations will happen serendipitously, in an informal, unexpected manner. You should be sensitive to hidden clues in conversations with your patients that may mask sexual concerns and follow up with open-ended questions."

Cultural influences on assessment

Little research in the literature addresses the sexuality issues of minorities [23]. Speculation regarding the reasons why minorities have been absent in sexuality research includes a possible mistrust of health care professionals because of negative past experience, or beliefs around sexuality that are more conservative [24]. This lack of research, in turn, makes it difficult for the nurse to be sure about when and how to speak to the patient, or to know whether he/she would even be a willing recipient of this information. A conversation about sexuality could be highly intrusive or embarrassing to the patient and partner, depending on their culture and what they believe is proper for discussion.

African american culture

Many elements influence the African American within the medical care system. Some of these components may include contextual factors (eg, lack of health insurance, few minority health care providers); religious and spiritual factors (faith in God); factors of general distrust in the medical system, which can lead to alternative medical practices; socioeconomic factors; social support; and empowerment factors [25,26]. Although these elements are related to health care in general, they must be kept in mind when making an attempt to assess and inform the patient about how his/her specific treatment will affect his/her sexuality.

Regarding discussing with a woman the sexual matters related to an illness like breast cancer, communication within the African American family may be minimal or absent, and grandparents, parents, aunts, and uncles may hesitate and be uncomfortable [23]. Wilmoth and Sanders [23], in their study of 16 African American women in a focus group setting, reported that the participants admitted that, in their culture, discussions about how their sexuality had changed during breast cancer treatment rarely happened, even among close female friends. They did verbalize interest in the sexual changes that had occurred in their bodies during treatment and said that they would prefer information in a one-on-one consultation, rather than in a group setting; they also said they thought they would be more open in a one-on-one conversation. However, they thought that a group setting was another suitable method for the nurse to provide information to them. One other study, with 12 African American heterosexual couples, revealed that, during the treatment process for breast cancer, sexual intimacy was difficult to maintain primarily because the husbands "were concerned about their wives' level of comfort with sexual intimacy, whereas women were more concerned about their physical appearance" [27]. Overall, the men were supportive, and reassured their wives that they would not leave them because of breast cancer. This study further mentioned the fact that these couples did not talk about sexuality issues with their health care provider, even though they felt it was important. These couples affirmed that some of their health care providers had been supportive, whereas others had not. Other reports stated that some African American women with breast cancer felt their providers were not sensitive to their particular needs and concerns [28,29].

Nurses providing assessment and intervention for African Americans must be aware of the hesitation of these patients to talk about sexuality issues within their own families; the exception seems to be the spouse or partner [27]. If hesitation exists, even within the family, the patient may not be willing to express concern about his/her sexuality, and it is paramount for the nurse to broach this subject first. One other issue is the "insider/outsider" dilemma (eg, whether or not the nurse is of the same ethnicity or culture as the patient); consequently, trust must be built and maintained by the nurse [26].

Asian American culture

East Asians can be of various cultural backgrounds (eg, Chinese, Japanese, Vietnamese, Cantonese, and so forth). For the most part, discussions of a sexual nature are essentially taboo in these families, and the older adults prefer not to talk about sex, often because they received an inadequate sex education [30]. Schools in Japan and Korea provide little in sex education, and sex is considered a private matter not to be discussed in public society [31,32]. East Asians have been found to be more conservative, have less sexual knowledge and experience, a later onset of sexual intercourse, and fewer sexual responses, when compared with other ethnic groups [33,34]. In Korea, parents are more tolerant of the sexual activities of their sons than of their daughters, and sex education emphasizes premarital virginity in girls. Premarital sexual activity is frowned on for both boys and girls, but a girl's premarital sexual activity is definitely viewed as a negative [35]. In general, health care professionals also shy away from discussing sexuality [36].

Reports in the literature acknowledge that Asian women have lower cancer screening rates than their Caucasian counterparts, which is thought to be partly because of fear or embarrassment, lack of time and money, and language limitations [37]. Acculturation (the process that occurs when a person moves to another culture and attempts to integrate into the new culture by taking characteristics and values of the new culture into his/her personality and self-identity) has also been noted to be a factor in cancer screening behaviors. In a study done by Woo and Brotto [38] with Euro-Canadian (n = 86) and East Asian (n = 78) women, the Canadian women had a significantly higher rate of Pap testing than the East Asian women. The Canadians were also found to be more knowledgeable about sex and to have a higher level of sexual functioning and a broader repertoire of sexual activities. The East Asian women cited embarrassment as a barrier to Pap testing; however, if more sexually permissive, they tended to be more likely to have had a Pap test. Acculturation to western culture was found to relate significantly to greater sexual desire. If the East Asian woman maintained strong ties to her culture, increasing mainstream acculturation did little to liberalize her sexual attitudes. But if she did relinquish her heritage culture to a certain degree, increasing exposure to North American culture led to more liberal sexual attitudes, and these women had higher Pap testing rates [38].

For the nurse with an East Asian patient, it must be ascertained whether or not this patient is a first-generation Asian and whether or not he/she has acculturated to this country. If embarrassment is associated with a simple Pap test, discussion of the patient's sexuality or sexual relationship may also cause embarrassment. Ishida [37] reported that Chinese women preferred information through the mail and not by telephone, and many Asian groups (Asian Indian, Chinese, Filipino, Japanese, Korean, and Vietnamese) showed little interest in an educational class format to acquire information. Consequently, the nurse should attempt to provide a one-on-one encounter with the patient for provision of information regarding sexuality issues, which provides privacy and decreases the potential for embarrassment.

Hispanic culture

Hispanics include primarily those persons from Mexico, Central and South America, Puerto Rico, and Cuba, and about 8% from other Spanish-speaking countries [39]. Social networks that include family and friends can be instrumental and a positive factor when providing medical care because they usually are involved in visits to the doctor and in the treatment that is to be delivered [40]. Because family involvement is valued and important to this culture, health care may be discussed and decided on by more than just the patient and partner. They may, however, be averse to seeking out medical care when an illness encompasses something involving sexuality. Adams and colleagues [41] report that "women have presented with long-standing gynecologic symptoms, such as bleeding after intercourse, which they were too embarrassed to bring to the attention of a health care provider." Hispanic women have a 7.3 times greater incidence of cervical cancer than Caucasian women, which may be because of a younger age at first intercourse. Overall, Hispanics are also reluctant to share marital problems that are caused by sexuality issues [41].

Traditionally, the Hispanic woman has been respected and is known to have a strong relationship with her children. Even after children are grown, this woman remains loving, caring, and nurturing [41]. On the other hand, in this culture, the male has created a submissive, self-relinquishing female who is fixated on procreation, and is necessarily devoted to her spouse and children [42]. Often, though, her strong dedication to family has put her own personal needs secondary to her family, with resultant delays in medical treatment for her own ailments.

In today's society, level of acculturation may significantly impact these populations' traditional views of femininity and machismo; individuals less acculturated respond differently than those who hold more "western" views [41]. The nurse may need to be somewhat more assertive, although not invasive, with the Hispanic population because of their shyness and reluctance to discuss sexuality issues with a health care provider, especially one who is not from within their own culture. Gentle persuasion may be appropriate for the nurse to be able to provide a good quality of education related to the illness and its impact on sexual function.

Summary

When assessing the patient and partner for issues or concerns relating to their sexuality, the nurse must not be more interested in finding treatment options than in normalizing the fact that they each have these issues. Help for these patients and partners is needed to find the causes of low order sexual functioning and to offer treatment options so they can have a better sense of their own sexuality and a more meaningful sex life. Recognition of a patient's entire sense of his/her own sexuality along with patient-centered goals acknowledges individual differences in sexual function. If the person is not troubled by a poor sexual performance, then he/she does not have a problem. During assessment and intervention planning, alternative sexual activities may be suggested; however, these may not be satisfying. Feelings of disappointment, failure, and distress may arise when none of the suggested strategies are helpful, and these feelings cannot be ignored. Essentially, no treatment program is 100% successful, and some patients and partners simply may not benefit from any treatment option.

References

[1] Huber C, Ramnarace T, McCaffrey R. Sexuality and intimacy issues facing women with breast cancer. Oncol Nurs Forum 2006;33(6):1163–7.

[2] Katz A. The sounds of silence: sexuality information for cancer patients. J Clin Oncol 2005; 23(1):238–41.

[3] Shell J. Impact of cancer on sexuality. In: Otto S, editor. Oncology nursing. 4th edition. St. Louis (MO): Mosby—Year Book, Inc.; 2001, p. 835–58.

[4] Wilmoth MC. Life after cancer: what does sexuality have to do with it? Oncol Nurs Forum 2006;33(5):905–10.

[5] Hughes MK. Sexuality and the cancer survivor. Cancer Nurs 2000;23(6):477–82.

[6] Wilmoth MC, Ross JA. Women's perception: breast cancer treatment and sexuality. Cancer Pract 1997;5(6):353–9.

[7] Feldman-Stewart D, Brundage M, Hayter C, et al. What questions do patients with curable prostate cancer want answered? Med Decis Making 2000;20(1):7–19.

[8] Bourgeois-Law F, Lotocki R. Sexuality and gynecological cancer: a needs assessment. Can J Hum Sex 1999;8:231–40.

[9] Hordern A. Intimacy and sexuality for the woman with breast cancer. Cancer Nurs 2000; 23(6):230–6.

[10] Kneece JC. Helping your mate face breast cancer. 5th edition. Columbia (SC): Educare Publishing; 2003.

[11] Ericksen JA, Steffen S. Kiss and tell: surveying sex in the twentieth century. Cambridge (MA): Harvard University Press; 1999.

[12] Haffner DW. Sexuality and scripture. Contemporary Sexuality 2004;38(1):7–10.

[13] Hyde J, DeLamater J, Byers E. Understanding human sexuality—Canadian edition. Toronto: McGraw Hill Ryerson; 2001.

[14] Rathus S, Nevid J, Ficher-Rathus L. Human sexuality in a world of diversity. 4th edition. Toronto: Allyn and Bacon; 2000.

[15] Carpenito-Moyet LJ. Nursing diagnosis: application to clinical practice. 10th edition. Philadelphia: Lippincott Williams and Wilkins; 2004.

[16] Annon J. The behavioral treatment of sexual problems. Honolulu (HI): Enabling Systems; 1974.

[17] Mick J, Hughes M, Cohen M. Sexuality and cancer: how oncology nurses can address it BETTER [abstract]. Oncol Nurs Forum 2003;30(Suppl 2):152–3.

[18] Spaulding S. No patient assessment is complete without asking one simple question. ONS News 2006;21(9):6.

[19] Rosen RC, Riley A, Wagner G, et al. The international index of erectile function (IIEF): a multidimensional scale for assessment of erectile dysfunction. Urology 1997;49(6): 822–30.

[20] Bruner DW, Boyd CP. Assessing sexuality. Cancer Nurs 1999;22(6):438–47.

[21] Mallinger JB, Griggs JJ, Shields CG. Patient-centered care and breast cancer survivors' satisfaction with information. Patient Educ Couns 2005;57(3):342–9.

[22] Sanders S, Pedro LW, Bantum EO, et al. Couples surviving prostate cancer: long-term intimacy needs and concerns following treatment. Clin J Oncol Nurs 2006;10(4):503–8.

[23] Wilmoth MC, Sanders LD. Accept me for myself: African American women's issues after breast cancer. Oncol Nurs Forum 2001;28(5):875–9.

[24] Haynes MA, Smedley BD. The unequal burden of cancer: an assessment of NIH research and programs for ethnic minorities and the medically underserved. Washington, DC: National Academy Press; 1999.

[25] Jenkins R, Schover LR, Fouladi RT, et al. Sexuality and health-related quality of life after prostate cancer in African-American and white men treated for localized disease. J Sex Marital Ther;30(2):79–93.

[26] Wilmoth MC, Narine L. African American women and cancer. In: Hassey Dow K, editor. Nursing care of women with cancer. St. Louis (MO): Mosby Elsevier; 2006, p. 433–43.

[27] Morgan PD, Fogel J, Rose L, et al. African American couples merging strengths to successfully cope with breast cancer. Oncol Nurs Forum 2005;32(5):979–87.

[28] Ashing-Giwa K, Ganz P. Understanding the breast cancer experience of African American women. J Psychosoc Oncol 1997;15(2):19–35.

[29] Moore RJ. African American women and breast cancer: notes from a study of narrative. Cancer Nurs 2001;24(1):35–42.

[30] Bhugra D, de Silva R. Sexual dysfunction across culture. Int Rev Psychiatry 1993;5:243–52.

[31] Kameya Y. How Japanese culture affects the sexual functions of normal females. J Sex Marital Ther 2001;27:151–2.

[32] Youn G. Perceptions of peer sexual activities in Korean adolescents. J Sex Res 2001;38: 352–60.

[33] Cain VS, Johannes CB, Avis NE, et al. Sexual functioning and practices in a multi-ethnic study of midlife women: baseline results from SWAN. J Sex Res 2003;40:266–76.

[34] Brotto LA, Chik HM, Ryder AG, et al. Acculturation and sexual function in Asian women. Arch Sex Behav 2005;34(6):613–26.

[35] Youn G. Sexual activities and attitudes of adolescent Koreans. Arch Sex Behav 1996;25(6): 629–43.

[36] Chan DW. Sex misinformation and misconceptions among Chinese medical students in Hong Kong. Arch Sex Behav 1986;19(1):73–93.

[37] Ishida DN. Asian women and cancer. In: Hassey Dow K, editor. Nursing care of women with cancer. St. Louis (MO): Mosby Elsevier; 2006. p. 444–58.

[38] Woo JST, Brotto LA. Cancer-screening behaviors, attitudes towards sexuality, and acculturation. Report from Society for Sex Therapy and Research Annual Meeting Atlanta (GA). 2007.

[39] U.S. Department of Commerce Bureau of the Census. The Hispanic population in the United States: March 1988 (advance report). Series P-20, No. 431. Washington, DC: U.S. Government Printing Office; 1988.

[40] Velez-Barone G. Latino women and cancer. In: Hassey Dow K, editor. Nursing care of women with cancer. St. Louis (MO): Mosby Elsevier; 2006. p. 472–81.

[41] Adams J, DeJesus Y, Trujillo M, et al. Assessing sexual dimensions in Hispanic women: development of an instrument. Cancer Nurs 1997;20(4):251–9.

[42] Diaz-Guerrero R. Psychology of the Mexican: culture and personality. Austin (TX): University of Texas Press; 1975.

ELSEVIER
SAUNDERS

Nurs Clin N Am 42 (2007) 697–703

NURSING
CLINICS
OF NORTH AMERICA

Index

Note: Page numbers of article titles are in **boldface** type.

Moving?

Make sure your subscription moves with you!

To notify us of your new address, find your **Clinics Account Number** (located on your mailing label above your name), and contact customer service at:

E-mail: elspcs@elsevier.com

800-654-2452 (subscribers in the U.S. & Canada)
407-345-4000 (subscribers outside of the U.S. & Canada)

Fax number: 407-363-9661

Elsevier Periodicals Customer Service
6277 Sea Harbor Drive
Orlando, FL 32887-4800

*To ensure uninterrupted delivery of your subscription, please notify us at least 4 weeks in advance of move.

1. Publication Title	2. Publication Number	3. Filing Date
Nursing Clinics of North America	5 9 8 - 9 9 6 0	9/14/07

4. Issue Frequency	5. Number of Issues Published Annually	6. Annual Subscription Price
Mar, Jun, Sep, Dec	4	$116.00

7. Complete Mailing Address of Known Office of Publication (Not printer) (Street, city, county, state, and ZIP+4)

Elsevier Inc.
360 Park Avenue South
New York, NY 10010-1710

Contact Person
Stephen Bushing

Telephone (Include area code)
215-239-3688

8. Complete Mailing Address of Headquarters or General Business Office of Publisher (Not printer)

Elsevier Inc., 360 Park Avenue South, New York, NY 10010-1710

9. Full Names and Complete Mailing Addresses of Publisher, Editor, and Managing Editor (Do not leave blank)

Publisher (Name and complete mailing address)

John Schrefer, Elsevier, Inc., 1600 John F. Kennedy Blvd. Suite 1800, Philadelphia, PA 19103-2899

Editor (Name and complete mailing address)

Alexandra Gavenda, Elsevier, Inc., 1600 John F. Kennedy Blvd. Suite 1800, Philadelphia, PA 19103-2899

Managing Editor (Name and complete mailing address)

Catherine Bewick, Elsevier, Inc., 1600 John F. Kennedy Blvd. Suite 1800, Philadelphia, PA 19103-2899

10. Owner (Do not leave blank. If the publication is owned by a corporation, give the name and address of the corporation immediately followed by the names and addresses of all stockholders owning or holding 1 percent or more of the total amount of stock. If not owned by a corporation, give the names and addresses of the individual owners. If owned by a partnership or other unincorporated firm, give its name and address as well as those of each individual owner. If the publication is published by a nonprofit organization, give its name and address.)

Full Name	Complete Mailing Address
Wholly owned subsidiary of	4520 East-West Highway
Reed/Elsevier, US holdings	Bethesda, MD 20814

11. Known Bondholders, Mortgagees, and Other Security Holders Owning or Holding 1 Percent or More of Total Amount of Bonds, Mortgages, or Other Securities. If none, check box ☐ None

Full Name	Complete Mailing Address
N/A	

12. Tax Status (For completion by nonprofit organizations authorized to mail at nonprofit rates) (Check one)
The purpose, function, and nonprofit status of this organization and the exempt status for federal income tax purposes:
☐ Has Not Changed During Preceding 12 Months
☐ Has Changed During Preceding 12 Months (Publisher must submit explanation of change with this statement)

PS Form 3526, September 2006 (Page 1 of 3 (Instructions Page 3)) PSN 7530-01-000-9931 PRIVACY NOTICE: See our Privacy policy in www.usps.com

13. Publication Title	14. Issue Date for Circulation Data Below
Nursing Clinics of North America	September 2007

15. Extent and Nature of Circulation			Average No. Copies Each Issue During Preceding 12 Months	No. Copies of Single Issue Published Nearest to Filing Date
a. Total Number of Copies (Net press run)			3600	3600
b. Paid Circulation (By Mail and Outside the Mail)	(1)	Mailed Outside-County Paid Subscriptions Stated on PS Form 3541. (Include paid distribution above nominal rate, advertiser's proof copies, and exchange copies)	2265	2197
	(2)	Mailed In-County Paid Subscriptions Stated on PS Form 3541 (Include paid distribution above nominal rate, advertiser's proof copies, and exchange copies)		
	(3)	Paid Distribution Outside the Mails Including Sales Through Dealers and Carriers, Street Vendors, Counter Sales, and Other Paid Distribution Outside USPS®	604	684
	(4)	Paid Distribution by Other Classes Mailed Through the USPS (e.g. First-Class Mail®)		
c. Total Paid Distribution (Sum of 15b (1), (2), (3), and (4))			2869	2881
d. Free or Nominal Rate Distribution (By Mail and Outside the Mail)	(1)	Free or Nominal Rate Outside-County Copies Included on PS Form 3541	87	74
	(2)	Free or Nominal Rate In-County Copies Included on PS Form 3541		
	(3)	Free or Nominal Rate Copies Mailed at Other Classes Mailed Through the USPS (e.g. First-Class Mail)		
	(4)	Free or Nominal Rate Distribution Outside the Mail (Carriers or other means)		
e. Total Free or Nominal Rate Distribution (Sum of 15d (1), (2), (3) and (4))			87	74
f. Total Distribution (Sum of 15c and 15e)			2956	2955
g. Copies not Distributed (See instructions to publishers #4 (page #3))			644	645
h. Total (Sum of 15f and g)			3600	3600
i. Percent Paid (15c divided by 15f times 100)			97.06%	97.50%

16. Publication of Statement of Ownership

☑ If the publication is a general publication, publication of this statement is required. Will be printed in the December 2007 issue of this publication. ☐ Publication not required.

17. Signature and Title of Editor, Publisher, Business Manager, or Owner

[signature] Date September 14, 2007

Stephen Fenucci - Executive Director of Subscription Services

PS Form 3526, September 2006 (Page 2 of 3)